DATE DUE

NO 17 '05			
DE 19 '05			
MAR 07 2011			
P			
E			

ABOUT THE AUTHOR

R. Eric Oestmann, Ph.D., M.S., P.T., earned his Doctorate in Health Services Administration from Southwest University in New Orleans, Louisiana. He earned a Masters degree in Physical Therapy from the University of South Dakota in Vermillion, South Dakota. Prior to that, he earned a Bachelors degree in Composite Physical Science from Black Hills State University.

Dr. Oestmann has a diversity of career experiences including six years in the United States Air Force; eight years of physical therapy practice in hospital, sports medicine, home health, private practice, and nursing home settings; healthcare administration experience; and six years of adjunct faculty teaching for Black Hills State University, Keller Graduate School of Management and Capella University.

Dr. Oestmann has self-published licensure and certification study guides and software for physical therapists, physical therapy assistants, occupational therapists, occupational therapist assistants, and athletic trainers. He has also published and presented continuing education materials to a variety of healthcare related disciplines. Currently, Dr. Oestmann is traveling throughout the country performing healthcare management consulting for Reo Healthcare Consulting, based on his doctoral dissertation, "Mutual Expectation Method Of Motivation™." He also continues his writing career with the production of "Proven Therapeutic Exercise Techniques" for Charles C. Thomas Publisher.

Dr. Oestmann lives in the beautiful Black Hills of South Dakota. He can be contacted at Reo Healthcare Consulting website, *www.reohealthcareconsulting.com.*

PROVEN THERAPEUTIC EXERCISE TECHNIQUES

Best Practices for Therapists and Trainers

By

R. ERIC OESTMANN, PH.D., M.S., P.T.

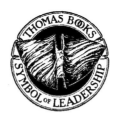

CHARLES C THOMAS • PUBLISHER, LTD.
Springfield • Illinois • U.S.A.

CHARLES C THOMAS • PUBLISHER, LTD.
2600 South First Street
Springfield, Illinois 62704

© 2004 by CHARLES C THOMAS • PUBLISHER, LTD.

ISBN 0-398-07514-X

Library of Congress Catalog Card Number: 2004045975

With THOMAS BOOKS *careful attention is given to all details of manufacturing and design. It is the Publisher's desire to present books that are satisfactory as to their physical qualities and artistic possibilities and appropriate for their particular use.* THOMAS BOOKS *will be true to those laws of quality that assure a good name and good will.*

Printed in the United States of America
GS-R-3

Library of Congress Cataloging-in-Publication Data

Oestmann, R. Eric.
    Proven therapeutic exercise techniques : best practices for therapists
and trainers / by R. Eric Oestmann.
        p.   cm.
    Includes bibliographical references and index.
    ISBN 0-398-07514-X (pbk.)
    1. Exercise therapy. I. Title.

RM725.O476 2004
615.8'2–dc22
                                                        2004045975

PREFACE

There are numerous books written on therapeutic exercise. Some specify unique techniques such as Pilates or Tai Chi, whereas others are extremely generic listing every possible exercise imaginable. The problems with both genres of exercise books are simple. If specific, they do not allow for eclectic exercise techniques and often require specialized equipment. If generic, they are not specific enough to be effective, nor efficient.

Health care professionals today are under constant financially based pressures to provide the most effective treatment in the most efficient time frame. Outcomes are vitally important. Financial savings are even more important as third party payers provide fuel for the health care economy. Therefore, effective outcomes with efficient costs are only possible within an exercise research basis.

While there are several professional journals and magazines that routinely contain information on exercise research, few practitioners have time to peruse them let alone learn the techniques and apply them correctly. Thus, the reason for creating this book is to review the past 20 years of research on therapeutic exercises and combine that knowledge base with over 8 years of clinical practice in order to provide a focused, yet eclectic book of therapeutic exercise for health care practitioners, especially physical therapists, physical therapy assistants, and athletic trainers.

The advantages of this book are obvious. Only those exercises that are researched and clinically proven to be effective and efficient will be found in this book. It simply saves the practitioner the time of performing independent research, participating in continuing education, and applying trial/error based learning. It saves the patient and their third party payers time and money as well.

While healthcare practitioner income is dependent on the number and length of treatments, gone are the days when we could just put a patient in the gym for an hour or two several times a week for an indefinite period of time. Third party payers are widely applying "Optimal Recovery Guidelines" (ORG) for certain diagnoses. These limitations require a focused treatment approach and the latest efficacious methods used. Those who hold steady to the practices of the past will soon become extinct.

Therefore, the format of this book is to provide empirical and research based exercises proven to work for a variety of diagnoses and conditions. Thus, only the absolutely "best" and most effective exercises are included in this book. It does not mean there are no other exercises to alleviate the conditions herein contained. It simply means that these have research data to back their efficacy and empirical evidence to support them. Pictures detail the correct exercise techniques along with descriptions of how they are to be performed.

Therapeutic exercise is the treatment mainstay of physical therapists, physical therapy assistants, and athletic trainers among other healthcare professionals. As I have discussed earlier in the preface, current therapeutic exercise books are either too specific or too general to be of significant benefit in today's healthcare environment. That environment, of course, being one controlled by third party payers and the "Optimal Recovery Guidelines" that often specifies a limited number of treatments per diagnosis regardless of outcomes. Therefore, this book has been specifically designed to provide "Proven" therapeutic exercise techniques for certain medical conditions in order to maximize effectiveness in a minimal amount of time.

These exercise techniques are "Proven" by researching over 20 years of MEDLINE and CINAHL databases for research articles related to therapeutic exercises yielding positive outcomes. This process has been an ongoing process as the proven therapeutic exercise research is correlated with over 8 years of clinical practice as a physical therapist. In fact, when I first started this process of creating a database of efficacious therapeutic exercises in 1995, I searched the research articles as far back as the 1950's. A unique finding occurred when I realized that the research "wheel" has a tendency to be reinvented nearly every 15 to 20 years.

By this I mean that there are research articles in the 1950's that have largely been reproduced in the 1970's and again in the 1990's with similar results. While many attribute this to good inter-rater reliability and validity, it simply reinforces the validity of limiting research to what has been done in the past 20 years. Furthermore, most current research references point to the previous data and works available. Thus, the reason for concentrating on the past 20 years of published and peer-reviewed research is established.

What has resulted from this combination of published research being confirmed or denied through clinically empirical findings is a system of effective and efficient therapeutic exercise intervention for any stage of patient injury. While other therapeutic exercise techniques may be effective for the conditions herein contained, we feel the ones in this book are the most focused and yield the outcomes desired in a minimum amount of treatment time.

Therapeutic exercise techniques are recommended accordingly by general tissue(s) involved; specific diagnosis; stage of injury, (i.e. acute, sub-acute, and chronic). Pictures and descriptions of efficacious therapeutic exercise techniques are included in each section and referenced accordingly at the end of each chapter. The final section of the book contains information on massage and joint mobilization/manual therapy among other special interest areas that are not often found in other therapeutic exercise texts.

It would be presumptuous to assume that we can provide specific exercise recommendations that are backed up with research data for every musculoskeletal diagnosis contained in the ICD-9 code book. However, we have covered a substantial number of diagnoses that are referred to physical therapists, physical therapy assistants, athletic trainers, and other rehab professionals.

Throughout this text, we have chosen to limit the number of exercises between 6 and 8. There are great reasons for this. First, is the fact that a home exercise program is nearly always appropriate for patients in the present healthcare environment. Second, is the fact that patient compliance with home exercise programs is only 50 percent with 6 to 8 exercises. The compliance rate goes down exponentially with an increasing number of home exercises. In fact, research has show that patient compliance drops to less than 10 percent for home exercise programs of 12 exercises or more.

In addition, I firmly believe in an integrated or eclectic treatment approach for all patients. It is rare that a patient will health effectively and efficiently when just one treatment is applied. This is precisely why we have recommended adjuncts to the proven therapeutic exercises that may include, modalities, joint mobilizations and manual therapy, massage, etc. These are only suggestions. Of course the clinician must always apply their own judgment in determining which suggestions are applicable and which are not.

In this book we assume the reader has the baseline knowledge of pertinent anatomy, joint mechanics, and muscle function/innervation for the region of the body to be treated. For quick reference we have included a short summary of anatomical information in Appendix 1. A chart listing normal ranges of motion for the body joints is also included in Appendix 2. In addition, we assume the reader is skilled and trained in differential diagnosis.

It is also important to remember that this is not a book of protocol. It is NOT a cook book. Subsequently, it is vitally important for the clinician to determine if any, part, or all of the "proven" exercises apply to the particular patient being treated before proceeding. Patient condition, goals, and response to treatment should be the obvious deciding factors in the choice of treatment intervention.

Disclaimer: Every treating clinician must rely on sound clinical judgment and evaluation findings when developing specific patient treatment plans.

This author wishes to extend a special thanks to my family and Mr. Michael Payne Thomas of Charles C Thomas, Publisher who have been supportive and helpful in this venture.

Eric Oestmann

"Tell me and I will forget. Show me and I may remember. But, involve me and I will understand." Confucius

The organization, research summaries and pictures in this book are all designed to do more than tell or show the reader. They are designed to involve you in the process of developing and implementing the most efficacious therapeutic exercise rehabilitation plan possible.

CONTENTS

PART I

INTRODUCTION

PART II

UPPER EXTREMITY PROVEN TECHNIQUES

PART III

LOWER EXTREMITY PROVEN TECHNIQUES

PART IV

SPINE PROVEN TECHNIQUES

PART V

SPECIAL CONSIDERATIONS PROVEN TECHNIQUES

PART VI

PROVEN JOINT MOBILIZATION TECHNIQUES

PART VII

PROVEN MASSAGE TECHNIQUES

PROVEN THERAPEUTIC
EXERCISE TECHNIQUES

Part 1

INTRODUCTION

Chapter 1

GENERAL THERAPEUTIC EXERCISE CONSIDERATIONS

I. **Therapeutic Exercise Preparations:** [1,3,4,5,6,10,12,14,18,21,24,26,27,29, 30,31,34,35,36,38,39,42,43,44,45,47,48,52,54,56,57,63,64,65,66,67,68,69,73,74,75,76,77,78,79,83, 85,86,87,91,93,94,97,98,106,108,109,110,111,115,118,120,123,125,126,130,132,135,137,138,139, 142,144,148,149,150,151]

   A. General Evaluation Considerations:
      1. The clinician should perform a detailed initial evaluation/assessment on each client prior to proceeding with the proven therapeutic exercise techniques.
        a. Medical records MUST first be extensively reviewed.
        b. Contraindications/Precautions MUST be noted.
        c. Physician orders (if applicable) MUST be obtained and followed.
        d. Musculoskeletal evaluation and differential diagnosis procedures can now commence.
      2. In addition to the preliminary information obtained it is important to:
        a. Determine the stage of the injury with each patient, (i.e., acute, subacute, or chronic) in order to determine what type of therapeutic exercise and/or modality treatments are most appropriate.
        b. Acute injuries generally last 2 to 4 days after occurrence and are characterized by pain, swelling, redness, heat, and decreased function.
          i. Therapeutic exercise treatment during the acute stage generally consists of passive range of motion to active assistive range of motion therapeutic exercise.

      ii. Modality treatments such as cryotherapy, ultrasound, and electrical stimulation are often indicated during the acute stage.

  c. Subacute injuries generally last between 10 to 17 days after the acute stage subsides, but may last up to 6 weeks after the initial occurrence. Inflammation, pain and loss of function are generally present but steadily improving in this stage.

      i. Therapeutic exercise treatment during the subacute stage generally consists of passive, active assistive, active, and even light resistive therapeutic exercise.

      ii. Modality treatments can include those used in acute injuries as long as they are not contraindicated and often extend to a variety of superficial and deep heat based treatments and/or traction during the subacute stage.

  d. Chronic injuries generally extend beyond 6 weeks time and chronic mild to moderate pain and/or inflammation may persist.

      i. Therapeutic exercise treatment during the chronic stage generally consists of ALL types of therapeutic exercise, (i.e., passive, active assistive, active, light resistive, progressive resistive, and sport/vocation specific).

      ii. Modality treatments are generally utilized less as the time of injury continues to progress. Again, modality treatments can include any that are not contraindicated during the chronic stage.

3. Next the clinician should determine the general type of injury or condition:

  a. Is it hypermobile?

  b. Is it hypomobile?

  c. Is it inflammatory?

  d. Is it a result of cumulative/repetitive trauma?

  e. Is it degenerative?

4. The fourth step is to determine the tissue(s) involved:

  a. Muscle.

  b. Ligament.

      c.   Nerve.

      d.   Vascular.

      e.   Bursa.

      f.   Bone.

      g.   Cartilage.

      h.   Joint/capsule.

5.   Fifth, the clinician should determine the desired goals/effects:

      a.   Increase strength.

      b.   Increase range of motion/mobility.

      c.   Increase flexibility.

      d.   Increase endurance.

      e.   Increase coordination.

      f.   Increase agility.

      g.   Increase balance.

      h.   Increase speed.

      i.   Increase stability.

      j.   Increase work/sport capacity.

      k.   Decrease pain.

      l.   Decrease muscle spasms.

B.   General Diagnosis Considerations:

1.   Once this is preliminary initial evaluation information is obtained, you should have enough information after physical inspection to determine the diagnosis.

      a.   Keep in mind many referring physicians may already have diagnosed your patient.

          i.   Even so, do NOT assume it is always 100 percent accurate.

      b.   Your specialized training and evaluation will sometimes lead you to conclude a different diagnosis than specified on a treatment order and it is important to recognize this for two primary reasons:

          i.   First, an accurate diagnosis is required for billing purposes. Often, multiple diagnoses apply and can extend "Optimal Recovery Guidelines" or ORG's that may be imposed by managed care organizations, insurance companies, and more frequently worker's compensation.

          ii.   Second, the correct diagnosis reduces the risk of potential litigation. As long as your objective evaluative findings support your concluding diagnosis, you should be on solid ground for treatment justification.

    2.   We will assume the reader of this text is competent in performing musculoskeletal evaluations and determining the appropriate diagnosis and course of treatment based on the goals at hand.

C.   General Treatment Considerations:

    1.   Although joint mobilization/manual therapy and massage techniques are covered in sections six and seven of this text, they are not necessarily required or necessary for every patient condition.

    2.   Modalities such as cryotherapy, hydrotherapy, ultrasound, electrical stimulation, traction, and the like are often important adjuncts to therapeutic exercise and serve to facilitate the healing process with many patients.

        a.   These and other modalities are thoroughly covered in another text recently printed by Charles C Thomas Publisher entitled, "Downer's 6th Edition, Therapeutic Techniques" by Eric Oestmann, PhD, PT and Ann Downer MS, PT available at *www.ccthomas.com.*

    3.   Although we have extensively reviewed 20+ years of research and correlated that research with empirical and clinically based best practices, every clinician MUST determine each exercise's applicability before blindly assigning them to a patient.

D.   General Patient Considerations:

    1.   If there is one thing that is probably the single most important ingredient for successful patient outcomes, it is the patient's level of MOTIVATION which directly corresponds to their COMPLIANCE.

        a.   Quite frankly, I have had patients who do not want to get better. These situations require an extra measure of tact and discipline by the treating clinician. However, in my doctoral dissertation, "Mutual Expectation Method Of Motivation – MEMOM™" I have learned an invaluable technique for motivating patients.

      b.   In a nutshell, the basis of MEMOM™ is to simply have the patient convey their expectations of treatment and return your expectations of compliance/recovery. Once this is established, it is much easier to sell your patients on the program you deem appropriate. It is as simple and as difficult as that.

      c.   For more information on the MEMOM™ method and seminar information, please contact Reo Healthcare Consulting at *www .reohealthcareconsulting.com*

II. **Therapeutic Exercise Documentation:**[3,4,21,24,34,42,43,44,47,51,62, 63,64,70,71,73,75,80,106,109,110,111,115,123,137,138]

    A.   Documentation is an absolute necessity in all healthcare evaluations and treatments.

    B.   While specific courses detail this, I feel it is important to summarize the most important aspects of documentation related to "Proven Therapeutic Exercise Techniques."

    C.   "MIFD":

       1.   *"M"ode* refers one of the following three types and their subtypes of therapeutic exercise:

          a.   Isometric (same length) resisted exercise occurs when the muscles contract without significant movement of the joint(s).

             i.   Most often it is applied directly by the treating therapist's hand holding a specific body segment instructing the patient to try and move the segment.

             ii.   Intensity of Isometric exercise is often recorded as "light," "medium," and "heavy."

          b.   Isotonic (same weight) resisted exercise consists of two types:

             i.   Concentric isotonic resisted exercise occurs when resistance is applied to a muscle as it contracts and shortens. This resistance can be manually applied by the therapist and graded the same as Isometric resisted exercise. Or, resistance can be applied by dumbbell weights, machine weights, or resistive bands/tubing most commonly.

      ii. Eccentric isotonic resisted exercise occurs when resistance is applied to a muscle as it contracts and lengthens. This resistance again can be manually applied by the therapist and graded the same as Isometric resisted exercise. Or, resistance can be applied by dumbbell weights, machine weights, or resistive bands/tubing most commonly. However, this type of Isotonic exercise does cause a greater stress on the cardiovascular system and higher risk of delayed onset muscle soreness than concentric exercise.

        iia. Plyometrics are a specific type of eccentric exercise commonly used in the athletic population that involves high velocity and high resistance. An example of plyometric exercise is progressive box jumping up/down using a variety of increasing heights.

c. Isokinetic (same speed) resisted exercise is based on hydraulic constant velocity with variable resistance working agonist and antagonistic muscles alternately (i.e., biceps – triceps).

      i. A selected speed of body segment movement is selected (i.e., 60 degrees per second through 180 degrees per second are most commonly used). As the client pushes and pulls harder the velocity stays constant but the torque increases.

      ii. This mode of resisted exercise is nearly always used in sport/work specific retraining. It is also frequently used in research studies as it is the most reliable method of measuring true strength and endurance in muscular tissues.

d. Open Chain exercise is used to identify exercise in which the extremity is allowed to move freely throughout space with or without resistance.

      i. An example of open chain exercise is the Bench Press.

e. Closed Chain exercise is used to identify exercise in which the extremity is fixed against an immovable object and the joint moves from the point of fixation.

        i.   An example of closed chain exercise is the Push Up.

  f.   Mode of exercise also refers to the position of the patient:

        i.   Supine (laying on the back).

        ii.   Prone (laying on the stomach).

        iii. Side lying (right or left).

  g.   Mode of exercise also refers to the body segment motion in the anatomical position of standing with the arms extended and palms facing up:

        i.   Abduction (away from the body).

        ii.   Adduction (toward the body).

        iii. External rotation (away from the body).

        iv. Internal rotation (toward the body).

        v.   Flexion (toward the head for extremities).

        vi. Extension (away from the head for extremities).

        vii. Pronation (palms down).

        viii. Supination (palms up).

        ix. Dorsiflexion (foot up).

        x.   Plantarflexion (foot down).

        xi. Inversion (ankle in).

        xii. Eversion (ankle out).

        xiii. Radial deviation (wrist out).

        xiv. Ulnar deviation (wrist in).

        xv. Protraction (outward movement).

        xvi. Retraction (inward movement).

        xvii. Elevation (upward movement).

        xviii. Depression (downward movement).

  h.   While most exercises are performed in the anatomical or muscle function patterns listed above, some conditions warrant the use of Proprioreceptive Neuromuscular Facilitation (PNF) patterns that involve combinations of planar movements. These provide an advanced coordination skill often used in patients suffering from a stroke or closed head injury. All PNF patterns have flexion and extension moments. The PNF patterns are as follows:

        i.   D1 Upper Extremity, the "Back Scratch" involves shoulder, elbow, wrist and finger flexion reaching diagonally across the chest and targeting the opposite shoulder blade from an extended and abducted position.

ii.   D2 Upper Extremity, the "Sword Out Of Pocket" involves shoulder, elbow, wrist and finger extension reaching diagonally from one hip and finishing the position as a knight would holding his sword, or a waiter holding a tray.

iii.   D1 Lower Extremity, the "Shin Scratch" involves hip, knee, ankle and toe flexion/dorsiflexion brushing the heel of the foot across the opposite shin. The hip also externally rotates in this pattern.

iv.   D2 Lower Extremity, the "Soccer Kick" involves hip and knee flexion with ankle and toe extension/plantarflexion, while the hip internally rotates and the leg kicks out as in the sport of soccer.

2.   "*I*"*ntensity* refers to the amount and quality of exercise resistance:

a.   Passive (PROM):

i.   When the patient is unable to actively move a body segment, the treating clinician moves it for them.

ii.   It is generally used in the acute stage of injury.

b.   Active Assistive (AAROM):

i.   When the patient is unable to actively move a body segment throughout the entire range of motion independently, the treating clinician assists them moving it.

ii.   It is generally used in the transition phases between acute and subactue injury status.

iii.   Some also qualify the amount of assistance as, "light," "moderate," and "significant."

c.   Active (AROM):

i.   When the patient is able to independently contract his muscles and move the body segment through the entire range of motion independently.

        ii.   The treating clinician does NOT assist in this task. It is generally used in the subacute phase of injuries.

   d. Resistive (RROM):

        i.   When a patient is able to begin re-strengthening activities in minimal pain, resistance (i.e., isometric, isotonic, or isokinetic) is applied by a variety of methods.

        ii.   This is generally reserved for treatment during the transition between subacute and chronic injury phases.

        iii. Weight and/or resistance measures such as foot pounds of torque are recorded.

        iv. It is also important to note the position of the clinician's hands on the body segment when performing manual resistance.

   e. Sport/Work Specific:

        i.   These are limited to the patients who require advanced therapeutic exercise training prior to sport/work return and are by their very nature sport/work specific.

        ii.   For example, if a college basketball player is injured it is usually part of rehabilitation to have them complete jumping and agility exercises specifically required of their sport. Many workers also perform functional capacity evaluations in which repetitive lifting, bending, stooping, etc. are performed prior to return.

3.   *"F"requency* refers to the number of exercise repetitions and sets of repetitions:

   a. The number of repetitions for each mode and its' intensity of therapeutic exercise is recorded.

   b. The number of sets of repetitions for each mode and intensity of therapeutic exercise is recorded.

        i.   For example, "3 sets of 10 repetitions of active left shoulder flexion in the supine position were performed with 1-2 minute breaks between sets."

   4.   *"D"uration* refers to the amount of time between exercise sets and/or repetitions, as well as the total length of treatment time:
        a.   Time frame is recorded in terms of how long the patient exercised or took for rest between sets of exercise.
             i.   For example, "3 sets of 10 repetitions of active left shoulder flexion in the supine position were performed with 1-2 minute breaks between sets for a total exercise time of 8 minutes."
        b.   In goal writing, duration also refers to the number of days, or weeks, or months during which an exercise program is to be performed.
   D.   Documenting functional outcomes is also critical in today's healthcare environment. Measurable data are often required by insurance companies and managed care organizations to determine average lengths of treatment per diagnosis in addition to the costs and outcomes associated with them.
        1.   Using the documentation example from above we would follow the MIFD protocol and add a functional component in the following example:
             a.   "3 sets of 10 repetitions of active left shoulder flexion in the supine position were performed with 1-2 minute breaks between sets for a total exercise time of 8 minutes in order for the patient to regain normal range of motion to perform required overhead work activities."
III.   **Specific Resistance Exercise Regimens with Research Efficacy:**[3,4,21,24,34,43,44,45,47,52,54,64,66,67,68,70,74,106,115,123,151]
   A.   *Brief Maximal Isometric Exercise:*
        1.   Hettinger and Muller developed this technique in the 1950's in which the patient performs a single isometric contraction of the muscle to be strengthened against manual resistance. The contraction is held 5 to 6 seconds and done once a day, 5 to 6 times per week.
   B.   *Brief Repetitive Isometric Exercise (BRIME):*
        1.   A modification on Hettinger and Muller's original study, it consists of 5 to 10 brief isometric contractions of the muscle to be strengthened against manual resis-

tance. The contractions are held 5 to 6 seconds and done once a day, 5 to 6 times per week.

C. *Multiple Angle Isometrics:*
1. Davies protocol consists of 10 sets of 10 repetitions of 10 second duration isometric contractions of the muscle to be strengthened against manual resistance every 10 degrees in the range of motion.

D. *DeLorme Technique:*
1. DeLorme developed the term progressive resistive exercise to detail his isotonic strengthening program in which the patient determines a 10 repetition maximum. This is the maximum amount of weight isotonically moved in 10 repetitions. The patient then performs 10 repetitions at 50 percent of the 10 rep maximum; 10 repetitions at 75 percent of the 10 rep maximum; and 10 repetitions at 100 percent of the 10 rep maximum. Three bouts of each exercise are performed three times per week and the 10 repetition maximum is tested and increased weekly.

E. *Oxford Technique:*
1. Developed by Oxford, this program is performed opposite of DeLorme's. The 10 repetition maximum is determined the same way. However, the patient performs 10 repetitions at 100 percent of the 10 rep maximum first; then performs 10 repetitions at 75 percent of the 10 rep maximum; and finally 10 repetitions at 50 percent of the 10 rep maximum. Again, three bouts of each exercise are performed three times per week and the 10 repetition maximum is tested and increased weekly.

F. *Daily Adjustable Progressive Resistance Exercise (DAPRE):*
1. Knight determines an initial working weight based on a 6 repetition maximum. The patient then performs 10 repetitions at 50 percent of the working weight; 6 repetitions at 75 percent of the working weight; and as many repetitions as possible at 100 percent of the working weight. If the final number of repetitions at 100 percent of the working weight is greater than 6, a new working weight is determined and provides the basis for the three sets of exercise sets for the next session.

Variations of this protocol continue to exist in the research literature with similar results.

G. *Isokinetic Strength Protocol:*
    1. In order to test strength/power, the research protocols call you to perform 4 to 8 repetitions of an exercise at 60 to 90 degrees per second speed.
    2. A deficit of 10 percent from non-dominant to dominant sides is normal.
        i.   For example, if a right hand dominant person performs 200 foot pounds of Peak Torque on the right shoulder and 180 foot pounds of Peak Torque on the left, it is considered normal.
        ii. However, if a right hand dominant person performs 200 foot pounds of Peak Torque on the right shoulder and 240 foot pounds of Peak Torque on the left, it is unbalanced with the right shoulder requiring more rehabilitation before return to sport or functional activity.
    3. Peak Torque is the measurement most commonly used to measure Isokinetic strength/power.
    4. In order to increase strength/power, the DeLorme, Oxford or DAPRE protocols are followed at 60 to 90 degrees per second speed.

H. *Isokinetic Endurance Protocol:*
    1. In order to test endurance, the research protocols call you to perform 15 to 30 repetitions of an exercise at 180 to 240 degrees per second speed.
    2. A deficit of 10 percent from non-dominant to dominant sides is normal.
        i.   Example: If a right hand dominant person performs 200 Watts of Total Work on the right shoulder and 180 Watts of Total Work on the left, it is considered normal.
        ii. However, if a right hand dominant person performs 200 Watts of Total Work on the right shoulder and 240 Watts of Total Work on the left, it is unbalanced with the right shoulder requiring more rehabilitation before return to sport or functional activity.

3. Total Work or Average Power are the measurements most commonly used to measure Isokinetic endurance.
4. In order to increase endurance, DeLorme, Oxford or DAPRE protocols are NOT used. Rather, a straight set or multiple sets of 15 to 30 repetitions at 180 to 240 degrees per second speed is followed.

I. *Circuit Training:*
1. Circuit training is generally used for global body fitness, strength and endurance training where a series of exercises, usually 15 to 20 in number are predetermined. Each exercise is performed for 40 seconds with 20 seconds of rest between exercises. The circuit is repeated if training beyond 15 to 20 minutes is required.

J. *Cardiovascular/Endurance Training:*
1. Normally this type of exercise protocol is performed between 70 and 90 percent of the Target Heart Rate, (e.g., 220-age = THR) for 20 to 30 minutes a minimum of 3 non-consecutive days per week.

K. Overload Principle:
1. All of the above techniques have been shown by double blinded research studies to be efficacious primarily because they are based on the overload principle which states, "In order to increase strength, a load that exceeds the metabolic capacity of the muscle must be used during the exercise.
2. The application of the overload principle in Isometric, Isotonic, and Isokinetic exercises leads to muscle hypertrophy (enlargement) and neuromuscular recruitment thereby increasing the strength of the muscle.

L. Delayed Onset Muscle Soreness (DOMS):
1. DOMS often occurs as a result of micro-breakage of the protein linkages between muscle fibers on a microscopic level. This is required for true strength and muscle hypertrophy to occur. The mild increase in pain and slight amount of swelling normally subsides within 24 to 48 hours. However, there is a fine line between DOMS and re-injury/trauma to the involved tissue. This should always be carefully documented and strengthening protocols adjusted to compensate for DOMS.

M. Overtraining/Overwork:
1. Overtraining/overwork is a phenomenon that actually causes temporary or permanent deterioration of strength as the result of over-exercising. Overtraining/overwork can generally be avoided if the intensity, duration, and progression of exercise fall within the parameters listed above. It is also important to note at least one day of rest per week is required to avoid overtraining/overwork. Preferably, there would be at least one day of relative rest between exercise sessions in order to avoid overtraining/overwork. Furthermore, overtraining/overwork is NOT the same thing as fatigue.
N. Fatigue:
1. Fatigue is a normal physiologic response of a muscle as it depletes its' supply of energy stores. This usually consists of depleting glucose, glycogen, oxygen and potassium which is replaced by lactic acid causing a burning sensation and muscle cramping or fatigue to be reported. Fatigue is normally short-lived and lasts a few seconds to a few minutes.

IV. **Specific Passive Stretching Regimens with Research Efficacy:**[3,4,5,12,20,33,34,36,38,42,47,51,64,76,87,98,104,118,123,126,144,148]
A. Stretching may be performed passively or in combination with Isometric active muscle contractions.
1. It is important to note that a muscle CANNOT be fully or effectively strengthened until it is of normal length.
2. It is also important to note that stretching is NOT Passive Range of Motion (PROM).
a. PROM is technically movement through the "free range" of motion.
b. Stretching pushes tissues beyond the free range to restore normal function.
B. Stretching Tips:
1. Warm up the area prior to stretching if there is no significant swelling.
2. ALWAYS apply a bit of joint distraction (traction) in order to reduce impingement pain of tissues during stretching.
3. ALWAYS stabilize the proximal body segment while moving the distal segment.

  a. For example, when stretching the elbow, make SURE to stabilize the shoulder.

 4. NEVER stretch over multiple joints as this will often overstretch the weaker joint/muscle.

 5. Due to passive insufficiency, distal muscles/joints should always be stretched before proximal ones.

C. Stretching Types:

 1. *Contract-Relax:*

  a. This technique is also referred to as "Muscle Energy" technique.

  b. It is incredibly effective for increasing range of motion fairly easy to teach patients.

  c. The process involves the therapist taking the tissue to the end range of motion and holding the body segment in that position while instructing the patient to contract, or push against, the therapist's hand . . . essentially performing an isometric contraction in which the muscle's origin and insertion are reversed.

  d. The isometric muscle contraction (which causes the Golgi tendon organ to fire thereby inhibiting muscle tension) is then released after a count of 2 to 5 seconds and the therapist proceeds to stretch tissues beyond "free range."

  e. This process is repeated 3 to 5 times with a break in between sets.

 2. *Contract-Relax-Contract:*

  a. This technique expands the Contract-Relax technique by adding an isometric contraction after the relaxation phase.

  b. The process is again repeated 3 to 5 times with breaks in between sets of 3 to 5.

  c. The research is conflicting as to which method (i.e., Contract-Relax or Contract-Relax-Contract is more effective).

   i. I have personally found both methods to be effective and efficient.

   ii. The determining factor for me is based strictly on patient tolerance and preference.

 3. *Reciprocal Inhibition:*

        a.   This type of stretching is also referred to as "Agonist Contraction."

        b.   It involves a type of self-stretching technique in which the patient contracts the muscle opposite of the one needing stretched.

           i.   For example, if the hamstrings are in need of elongation you would instruct the patient to contract the quadriceps and hold for a count of 15 to 30 seconds and repeat 3 to 5 times thereby stretching the hamstrings.

        c.   It is particularly useful if the patient does not tolerate manual (therapist) stretching especially in the early or acute stage of injury.

        d.   It is least effective when the patient is nearing normal range of motion.

    4.   *Static Prolonged:*

        a.   Passive range of motion is performed into tissue resistance.

        b.   The research indicates 3 to 5 sets of 15 to 30 second stretching force applied to a muscle is every bit as effective at lengthening the tissue as anything beyond this amount.

        c.   However, the patient must relax completely in order for the stretching procedures to be effective.

           i.   Most therapists and researchers agree that pain beyond a "7" on a Likert 0 to 10 Pain Rating Scale (0 = none and 10 = maximum), is counterproductive as automatic pain reflexes will kick in and contract tissue in order to attempt to protect itself.

           ii.   Ballistic or bouncing with stretching is an inappropriate stretching technique as it will also cause micro tearing of muscular tissues.

V. **Concept of Muscle Balance:**[34,47,51,62,63,64,109,110]

    A.   Before we dive right into the proven exercise techniques, it is essential to point out the concept of muscle balance:

        1.   Every joint in the body has a group of muscles, ligaments, and joint capsular tissue that holds it together.

        2.   If any one or more of these structures is out of balance it can create a predisposition for injury.

      3.   Conversely, trauma often disrupts this balance and pre-disposes it to further injury if not corrected.

   B.   One of the most overlooked aspects of any professional musculoskeletal treatment/rehabilitation program is muscle balance.

   C.   What is established by research is the fact that the major joints in the body follow a prescribed ratio of flexor to extensor muscle balance.

      1.   Anytime these strength ratios are imbalanced, pain and compromised healing is likely to result.

      2.   Most of these strength ratios are well researched and based on standard normal population groups: [11,16,24,28]

         a.   Cervical Flexors ⅔ as strong as Cervical Extensors.

         b.   Thoracic Extensors ⅔ as strong as 1 Thoracic Flexors.

         c.   Lumbar Flexors ⅔ as strong as 1 Lumbar Extensors.

         d.   Hamstrings ⅔ as strong as 1 Quadriceps.

   D.   Each minor joint in the body also follows certain flexor to extensor ratios, but with much less certainty.

      1.   Therefore, the clinician must carefully consider the balance of each joint, even minor ones, in order to minimize predisposition to injury after rehabilitation.

  VI. **Exercise Argot:**

   A.   The term "Argot" refers to the language of a specific profession or professional subset:

      1.   It is a concept I always teach with my first classes of college students.

      2.   Its' importance sets the tone for successful teaching of any topic.

   B.   Essentially, once the argot of a profession is learned it becomes a facilitating environment for learning.

      1.   For example, law students often struggle in the first semester of course work which is primarily due to the overwhelming amount of new terminology specific to law.

      2.   Medical students, physical therapy students, athletic training students, et cetera, all experience the same phenomenon.

         a.   It is more than just an over abundance of material to read and process and those who understand this concept and apply it early in their educational development nearly always succeed.

        b.   Those who do not understand the language of their particular course or professional WILL always struggle.

C.   Thus, one of the purposes of this introductory chapter is to detail the argot/language of proven therapeutic exercise techniques.

D.   With that in place, enjoy the remainder of this text.

Chapter 2

SUMMARY THERAPEUTIC
APPLICATION PEARLS

I. **General Therapeutic Exercise Contraindications:**[3,4,34,44,47,51,63,64,70,71,77,106,115,123,137]

   A. Common contraindications to active or passive exercise includes, but is not limited to: [12,14,19,26]
      1. Increased Inflammation.
      2. Unstable Cardio-Vascular Problems.
      3. Severe Osteoporosis.
      4. Ischemia/Peripheral Vascular Disease (PVD).
      5. Severe Pain Lasting More Than 24 Hours.
      6. Positive (+) Vertebral Artery Test for Cervical Spine Pathology.
      7. Positive (+) Homan's Test for Deep Vein Thrombosis.
      8. Bony Block.
      9. Significant Disruption To The Healing Process.
      10. Infection.
      11. Fracture.
      12. Hematoma's.
      13. Malignancy.

II. **General Therapeutic Exercise Precautions/Red Flags:**[3,4,34,44,47,51,63,64,70,71,77,106,115,123,137]

   A. It is critical to follow physician protocols regarding post surgical and post fracture care with their patients.
   B. These protocols ALWAYS supercede independent treatment plans and serve to protect the treating clinician from tort or malpractice legal actions.
   C. Red Flags for possible visceral pathology (i.e., cancer) include but are not limited to:[25]
      1. Weight Fluctuations.
      2. Inability To Sleep.
      3. Medications Are Required To Sleep.

       4.   Pain Becomes Worse With Walking.

       5.   Recent Fever Or Infection.

  D. Other Precautions include:

       1.   Delayed Onset Muscle Soreness (DOMS).

       2.   Overtraining/Overwork.

       3.   Severe Osteoporosis.

       4.   Degree of Ischemia/Peripheral Vascular Disease (PVD).

       5.   Steroid Use.

       6.   Age.

       7.   Avoiding Valsalva Maneuver.

III. **General Therapeutic Exercise Indications:** [3,4,34,44,47,51,63,64,70,71,77,106,115,123,137]

  A. Weakness.

  B. Pain.

  C. Low Endurance.

  D. Musculoskeletal Injury/Trauma.

  E. Decreased Joint Proprioreception.

  F. Decreased Range Of Motion.

  G. Decreased Flexibility.

  H. Decreased Circulation.

  I. Decreased Bone Density.

  J. Impaired Functional (Vocational/Avocational) Activities.

  K. Muscle Spasms.

  L. Progressive Degeneration.

  M. Swelling/Edema.

IV. **General Therapeutic Exercise Goals/Benefits:** [3,4,34,44,47,51,63,64,70,71,77,106,115,123,137]

  A. Increased Strength.

  B. Increased Range of Motion.

  C. Increased Flexibility.

  D. Increased Endurance.

  E. Increased Coordination.

  F. Increased Agility.

  G. Increased Balance.

  H. Increased Speed.

  I. Increased Stability.

  J. Increased Function.

  K. Decreased Pain.

  L. Decreased Muscle Spasms.

V. **Clinical Relevance Research Pearls:** [1,3,4,5,6,10,12,14,18,21,24,26,27, 29,30,31,34,35,36,38,39,42,43,44,45,46, 47,48,52,54,56,57,63,64,65,66,67,68,69,73,74,75,76,77,78, 79,83,85,86,87,91,93,94,97,98,106,108,109,110,111,115,118,120,123,125,126,130,132,135,137,138, 139,142,144,148,149,150,151]

A. It is very important to understand the overall goal of Therapeutic Exercise (TEX) is to have symptom free movement and function in the quickest amount of time possible.

B. In order to achieve this overriding goal of TEX, it is advantageous to apply the following research pearls of efficacy where appropriate.

C. GENERAL RESEARCH TEX PEARLS:

1. The proper sequence to increase range of motion and strengthen is:
   a. Joint Mobilizations first.
   b. Stretching second.
   c. Strengthening third.

2. Each joint needs 10 repetitions of full Range of Motion (Active or Passive) to provide minimal joint nutrition daily.

3. One day of bed rest takes 1 week of exercise to return prior muscle strength/function.

4. It takes 6 to 8 weeks to see true strength gains.

5. Short term increases in muscle strength (<6 weeks) are primarily due to increased synaptic transmission at the neuromuscular junction.

6. Wellness is a measure of Health and Fitness.

7. Fitness is a measure of Cardiorespiratory Capacity plus Muscle Endurance plus Muscle Strength plus Flexibility.

8. Motor Performance is a measure of Coordination plus Balance plus Power plus Agility plus Speed plus Reaction Time.

9. Motor Performance is an adjunct to Wellness.

10. To increase muscle endurance, perform high numbers of repetitions (>15) at low weight/resistance.

11. To increase muscle power, perform low numbers of repetitions (<10) at high weight/resistance.

12. Frenkel's exercises are specifically designed to improve coordination and skill.

     a.   They commonly include alternating heel slides, hip abduction/adduction, heels up the shin, marking time, walking sideways and tandem.

13. Strength gains during eccentric training have been shown to partially persist over 8 weeks of detraining.

14. Stretching hamstring muscles prior to strength testing has been shown to increase peak torque up to 25 percent.

15. Therapeutic exercise is often limited because of pain and joint shifting associated with open chain exercise, whereas weakness often limits closed chain exercise.
     a.   The solution to this problem is "Unloading" (i.e., closed chain exercise with a decrease in the patient's weight provided by self supporting harness or the patient lifting partially on a lat pull down machine or similar apparatus).

16. Exercise with patients who have Guillain-Barre or Multiple Sclerosis must consider fatigue and heat as 2 complications to exercise.
     a.   Consider early morning exercise in cool ambient air temperatures with frequent rest breaks to maximize effectiveness.

17. Range of motion should be initiated in burn patients as soon as possible as the position of comfort becomes the position of contracture without movement.

18. Exercise increases volume of muscle 20 percent, a factor to consider with patients who have Compartment Syndrome.

19. As you design an exercise program for geriatric patients a rule of thumb to follow is to consider what you can accomplish with a 20 year old patient and cut the intensity in half, and add double the rest breaks.

20. In general terms Cardiogenic pain causes decreased ventilation, decreased heart rate, and decreased blood pressure.

21. In general terms Peripheralgenic pain causes increased ventilation, increased heart rate, and increased blood pressure.

22. Adjuncts to therapeutic exercise include modalities:

a. Biofeedback/Myofeedback to increase or decrease muscle activity.
b. Electrical Stimulation to increase muscle activity or reduce pain.
c. Cryotherapy and/or Massage after exercise to decrease effects of DOMS.
d. Superficial or Deep Heat before exercise to increase blood flow, nerve transmission and increase flexibility.

23. Weight bearing exercise is essential for osteoporotic patients to build bone density.
   a. Therefore, closed chain exercises are essential for this population.
24. Weight bearing also increases joint proprioreception and increases co-contraction for neurologically impaired patients.
25. Anaerobic energy systems (Adenosine Tri-Phosphate and Creatine) are used with high intensity, short duration exercise less than 10 seconds.
26. Anaerobic glycolysis (Sugar) energy systems are used with high intensity, short duration exercise from 10 to 40 seconds.
27. Aerobic energy metabolism is predominately used with low intensity, long duration exercise exceeding 10 minutes in duration.
28. Allowing visual knowledge of results with exercise has been proven to increase peak torque as compared to exercise without knowledge of results.
   a. This is most effective in Isokinetic exercise applications.
29. Aquatic exercise should be performed in a pool at 86 degrees Fahrenheit or less in order to prevent dehydration and overheating.
30. Pregnant patients should avoid supine exercises after the first trimester secondary to decreased cardiac output in the supine position .
31. Pregnant patients should avoid deep flexion of joints secondary to increased Relaxin hormones and decreased ligament stability.

32. Exercises to avoid with musicians include:
    a.   Grip exercises.
    b.   Isolated hand and finger flexion exercises.
33. Aerobic exercise benefits patients with Fibromyalgia resulting in lower pain ratings.
34. Isometric exercise is generally indicated with acute injury even if swelling is present to prevent muscle atrophy as long as exercise does not increase swelling.
35. As patients age increases the number of Type II "Fast Twitch" muscle fibers decreases while Type I "Slow Twitch" fibers are largely unaffected.
    a.   Therefore, utilizing exercises that facilitate Type II "Fast Twitch" muscle fibers should be considered in exercise regimens for the geriatric population.
36. Maximum Heart Rate = 220 minus (-) age for land based exercise.
37. Maximum Heart Rate = 205 minus (-) age for aquatic based exercise.
38. Maximum Heart Rate = less than 140 beats per minute for pregnant persons.
39. Maximum Heart Rate = 170 to 175 beats per minute for people with Down's Syndrome.
40. Resting blood pressure greater or equal to $^{200}/_{100}$ mmHG contraindicates exercise.
41. Exercise blood pressure greater or equal to $^{240}/_{110}$ mmHG contraindicates exercise.
42. Resting heart rate greater than 130 beats per minute contraindicates exercise.
43. Exercise heart rate greater than 85 percent of Maximum Heart Rate contraindicates exercise.
44. Resting respiration greater than 45 breaths per minute contraindicates exercise.
45. Exercise respiration greater than 60 breaths per minute contraindicates exercise.

D. CARDIO/PULMONARY RESEARCH TEX PEARLS :
    1.   Patients on Beta Blockers, Ace Inhibitors and Calcium Channel Blockers generally have blunted blood pressure and heart rate responses to exercise.
    2.   Patients with COPD (Chronic Bronchitis, Emphysema, Cystic Fibrosis, Asthma and Bronchopulmonary Dys-

plasia) should not have their oxygen turned up during exercise or cardiac failure is likely.

3.   Normal blood pressure responses to exercise include: increased heart rate, increased systolic blood pressure, increased respiration and status quo or slightly decreased diastolic blood pressure.

4.   Patients lose 50 percent of their cardiovascular reserve with 4 days of bed rest.

5.   Patients with an Automatic Internal Cardiac Defibrillator (AICD) are NOT candidates for abdominal exercises.

6.   Patients with Diabetes Mellitus generally have blunted heart rate and blood pressure responses to exercise.

7.   Patients taking Cyclosporin generally have blood pressure responses greater than normal to exercise.

8.   Do NOT allow patients to lie supine after exercises because of poor lung ventilation/perfusion ratios and patients with congestive heart failure that will likely arrest because of overloading the right atrium with venous blood.

9.   Water aerobic exercises have been shown to decrease heart arrhythmias versus land based exercise with no difference in heart rate in comparing similar exercises.

10.   Avoid exercise within 1 to 2 hours after meals.

11.   Avoid upper extremity isometrics and Valsalva (holding breath) as this increases Intrathecal pressure and restricts heart performance.

E.   ORTHOPEDIC RESEARCH TEX PEARLS:

1.   Joint specific contraindications depend on surgical approach applicable to joint replacements most frequently from 8 to 12 weeks after surgery:

a.   Total Hip Replacement (THR) Posterior Lateral approach:
i.   NO hip flexion above 90 degrees.
ii.   NO hip adduction past neutral.
iii.   NO hit internal rotation past neutral.

b.   Total Shoulder Replacement (TSR) Anterior Lateral Approach:
i.   NO shoulder external rotation.
ii.   NO shoulder abduction.

   iii. NO shoulder extension.
2. Return to competition/work criteria discharge from therapy following knee injuries is:
  a. Ninety (90) percent strength of the uninvolved knee and successful functional testing.
  b. Sixty Six (66) percent is the ideal Hamstring to Quadriceps ratio before return to sport is allowed.
  c. Eighty (80) percent strength of the uninvolved knee is regarded as functional for those NOT involved in athletic competition.
3. Return to competition/work criteria following shoulder rotator cuff repair is:
  a. Eighty (80) percent strength of the uninvolved shoulder external rotators.
  b. Ninety (90) percent strength of the uninvolved shoulder internal rotators.
4. Shoulder exercises for internal and external rotation should be performed in the "Plane of the Scapula" (i.e., 30 degrees of abduction) to prevent wringing of the Supraspinatus.
5. The most appropriate time to begin progressive resistive exercise after joint replacement surgery is 6 weeks.
6. The minimum functional amount of knee flexion for patients with total knee replacements is 110 degrees.
7. The most common complication with total knee replacements is lack of full knee extension.
  a. The reason why full knee extension is so important after a total knee replacement involves a causative limp.
8. Isokinetic exercises at high speeds have been shown to decrease patellar-femoral pain secondary to Bernoulli's Principle which states, "Increased speed of fluid movement decreases surface pressure at the synovial fluid interface between patella and femur."
9. Backward walking/jogging has been shown to decrease patellofemoral pain.
10. Patellar taping prior to exercise decreases knee pain allowing increased Quadriceps loading in closed chain exercises.
11. The most appropriate muscles to concentrate on strengthening after an Anterior Cruciate Ligament

(ACL) deficiency are the Hamstrings and Plantarflexors.

    a.   These muscles limit anterior knee translation.

12. The most appropriate muscles to concentrate on strengthening after a Posterior Cruciate Ligament (PCL) deficiency are the Quadriceps.

    a.   These muscles limit posterior knee translation.

13. Patients with PCL injuries should avoid open chain hamstring work secondary to posterior Tibial translation until grafting is set or healed, usually 8 to 12 weeks after surgery.

14. Patients with ACL injuries should avoid open chain Quadriceps work secondary to anterior Tibial translation until grafting is set or healed, usually 8 to 12 weeks after surgery.

15. Patello-femoral pain is associated with Calcaneal Valgus, Forefoot Varus, tight Ilio-Tibial Band, Gastrocnemius and Hamstring muscles, and an increased "Q" Angle.

16. ACL reconstruction functional tests include:

    a.   Figure of 8 running and stair running functional tests are best correlated with function at the 3 month post operative mark.

    b.   Unilateral triple hop and stair hopple functional tests are best correlated with function/strength and stability of the knee at the 6 month post operative mark.

17. ACL rehabilitation should include a component of weight bearing closed chain exercise early in the process because it decreases ACL translation.

18. Osteochondritis Dissicans generally needs surgery to correct the problem, however in the interim clinicians should institute 4 way hip exercises (Hip Adduction, Abduction, Flexion and Extension) as well as Hamstring/Quadriceps co-contractions with the knee extended to maintain strength.

19. Normal pre-operative muscle strength generally occurs after 4 to 6 weeks arthroscopic surgery and 3 to 4 months ACL reconstruction.

Part 2

UPPER EXTREMITY
PROVEN TECHNIQUES

Chapter 3

PROVEN THERAPEUTIC EXERCISE TECHNIQUES – UPPER EXTREMITY

I. **General Upper Extremity Exercise Contraindications:**
    3,4,34,44,47,51,63,64,70,71,77,106,115,123,137

    A. Common contraindications to active or passive exercise in-
        cludes, but is not limited to: [12,14,19,26]
        1. Increased Inflammation.
        2. Unstable Cardio-Vascular Problems.
        3. Severe Osteoporosis.
        4. Ischemia/Peripheral Vascular Disease (PVD).
        5. Severe Pain Lasting More Than 24 Hours.
        6. Bony Block.
        7. Infection.
        8. Fracture.
        9. Malignancy.

II. **General Upper Extremity Exercise Precautions/Red
    Flags:** 3,4,34,44,47,51,63,64,70,71,77,106,115,123,137

    A. It is critical to follow physician protocols regarding post sur-
        gical and post fracture care with their patients.
    B. These protocols ALWAYS supercede independent treatment
        plans and serve to protect the treating clinician from tort or
        malpractice legal actions.
    C. Red Flags for possible visceral pathology (i.e., cancer) in-
        clude but are not limited to: [25]
        1. Weight Fluctuations.
        2. Inability To Sleep.
        3. Medications Are Required To Sleep.
        4. Pain Becomes Worse With Walking.
        5. Recent Fever Or Infection.
    D. Other precautions include:
        1. Delayed Onset Muscle Soreness (DOMS).
        2. Overtraining/Overwork.

      3. Severe Osteoporosis.
      4. Degree of Ischemia/Peripheral Vascular Disease (PVD).
      5. Steroid Use.
      6. Age.
      7. Avoiding Valsalva Maneuver.

III. **General Upper Extremity Exercise Indications:** [3,4,10,34,44,47,51,63,64,70,71,77,106,115,123,137]

    A. Common Diagnoses:
      1. Arthritis (Osteoarthritis and Rheumatoid Arthritis).
      2. Degenerative Joint Disease (DJD).
      3. Post Surgical Arthroscopies and Arthroplasties.
      4. Thoracic Outlet Syndrome/Thoracic Inlet Syndrome (TOS/TIS).
      5. Brachial Plexus Nerve Entrapment/Neuropathy.
      6. Ulnar Nerve Entrapment.
      7. Carpal Tunnel Syndrome.
      8. Cubital Tunnel Syndrome.
      9. Pain.
      10. Muscle Spasms.
      11. Muscle Strains.
      12. Ligament Sprains.
      13. Joint Dislocations.
      14. Cartilage Tears/Meniscus Lesions.
      15. Bursitis.
      16. Adhesive Capsulitis.
      17. Contusions.
      18. Muscle Atrophy/Weakness.
      19. Dequervain's Stenosing Tenosynovitis.
      20. Synovitis.
      21. Reflex Sympathetic Dystrophy.
      22. Tendonitis.
      23. Post Facture Care.
      24. Myositis.
      25. Sprengel's Deformity.
      26. Osteoporosis.

IV. **General Upper Extremity Exercise Goals/Benefits:** [3,4,34,44,47,51,63,64,70,71,77,106,115,123,137]

    A. Increased Strength.
    B. Increased Range of Motion.
    C. Increased Flexibility.

    D.   Increased Endurance.

    E.   Increased Coordination.

    F.   Increased Agility.

    G.   Increased Balance.

    H.   Increased Speed.

    I.   Increased Stability.

    J.   Increased Function.

    K.   Decreased Pain.

    L.   Decreased Muscle Spasms.

IV. **Upper Extremity Research Contributors:**[11,21,22,84,135,146]

    A.   This section is largely based on the research works by George Davies, Tab Blackburn, Mike Voight, Kevin Wilk and Steven Tippet.

        1.   They are experts in upper extremity rehabilitation and former or current affiliates with the North American Sports Medicine Institute.

    B.   These renowned therapists introduced me to the concept of muscle imbalances back in 1993.

        1.   What I learned from their research is the fact that muscle imbalances can occur from front to back (anteriorly to posteriorly) or right to left.

    C.   Muscle imbalances can result from a myriad of different reasons:

        1.   Dominant versus non-dominant sides.

        2.   Pain.

        3.   Incorrect strengthening and stretching exercises.

    D.   We are all familiar with the weight lifter at the gym who continuously works on the Biceps and Pectorals, and quadriceps, but who ignores the upper back muscles.

        1.   The result is a typical anterior muscle imbalance which rounds out the upper back into extreme kyphosis and often causes some type of shoulder dysfunction and/or impingement.

    E.   Another extremely common thing I encounter is the improper techniques people use when lifting weights and performing exercises.

        1.   The number one thing I see as a problem in this area is the fact that people perform exercises too fast.

            a.   This causes them to recruit ancillary muscles to complete the exercises.

2. The second thing I see as a problem in this area is the fact that people consistently tear up their Rotator Cuff by performing the Dumbbell Fly exercise above the level of the shoulder and NOT in the "Plane of the Scapula."

    a. This wrings out the Supraspinatus and cuts it on the Subacromial arch much the same way a rope becomes frayed as it dangles over a rocky ledge.

F. Due to the complex nature of the upper extremity, each of the following chapters are divided into the following:

1. Hypomobile Conditions and Proven Therapeutic Exercise Techniques.

2. Hypermobile Conditions and Proven Therapeutic Exercise Techniques.

3. Neurovascular Conditions and Proven Therapeutic Exercise Techniques.

4. Post Fracture/Surgical Conditions and Proven Therapeutic Exercise Techniques.

    a. The proven therapeutic exercises in each division may be applicable in more than one area depending on the diagnosis.

        i.   For example in the post fracture/surgical division, the hypomobile exercises are generally applicable in the early phase of rehabilitation.

        ii. Whereas, the hypermobile exercises are generally applicable in the later phases of post fracture/surgical rehabilitation.

    b. Therefore, it is imperative that the treating clinician review ALL of the Proven Therapeutic Exercises for each condition and fully evaluate the patient prior to initiating a custom rehabilitation program for a particular patient.

Chapter 4

SHOULDER & SHOULDER GIRDLE

I. **General Shoulder Considerations:** [11,21,22,23,34,40,47,64,71,90,102,109,110,113,117,119,140,143,146]

A. The shoulder is the MOST unstable joint in the body.

B. It is important to perform a complete musculoskeletal evaluation in order to determine the correct pathology and/or symptoms before proceeding with therapeutic exercise treatment.

C. One of the advantages with extremity evaluations is the fact that only one side is normally affected and the clinician may use the other side as a "normal" baseline.

    1. Keep in mind that a 10 percent strength differential is considered normal for the dominant hand side.

        a. For example, it would be considered normal in a right handed dominant individual to be 10 percent stronger on their dominant side.

D. It is important to exercise the Rotator Cuff muscles in the "Plane of the Scapula" which is defined as 30 degrees horizontal humeral abduction.

    1. This position is easily maintained by securing a pillow around the mid-section of the patient.

    2. If this position is not maintained during shoulder rehabilitation exercises the Supraspinatus becomes wringed or twisted with shoulder flexion and abduction in particular, thus cutting off the blood supply to the muscle and increasing the likelihood of necrosis and tissue injury.

E. Rotator Cuff non-surgical management advocated by McLaughlin:

    1. There are 4 reasons to be patient with non-surgical rehabilitation in the event of Rotator Cuff tears:

        a.   At least 25 percent of cadaver shoulders have a torn or degenerated Rotator Cuff.

        b.   More than 50 percent of patients with a ruptured Rotator Cuff recover spontaneously.

        c.   Accurate diagnosis can be difficult in the early painful period, which can lead to unnecessary surgery.

        d.   The results of early versus delayed surgical Rotator Cuff repairs are substantially the same.

    2.   In other words, give rehabilitation time to work.

        a.   In fact, most surgeons I have worked with prefer to wait 3 months or more before agreeing to operate, and there is good reason for this based on McLaughlin's work.

F.   Therapeutic exercise for balanced shoulder rehabilitation progression:

    1.   The "PRICE" principle applies for all shoulder rehabilitation that involves inflammation and/or trauma.

        a.   "P"rotection often means refraining from sport or activity.

            i.   It may also involve a sling such as a Kenny Howard style.

        b.   "R"est often means taking a break from activity.

            i.   Keep in mind this excludes range of motion that requires 10 repetitions daily to maintain joint nutrition.

        c.   "I"ce or cryotherapy will reduce pain and inflammation.

        d.   "C"ompression will also reduce pain and inflammation.

            i.   Ace compression wraps are commonly used for the shoulder.

        e.   "E"levation will prevent distal extremity edema and often involves laying supine or side lying on the uninvolved shoulder.

            i.   Sitting and standing should be minimized.

II. **Shoulder Imbalances:**[11,21,22,23,34,40,47,64,71,90,102,109,110,113,117,119, 140,143,146]

    A.   Range of motion imbalances occur in the shoulder complex which is made up of four anatomical and functional joints:

1. The Glenohumeral (GH) Joint:
   a. This tri-planar joint creates the majority of range of motion in the shoulder complex.
   b. This is the joint where the Rotator Cuff musculature attaches.
2. The Acromioclavicular (AC) Joint:
   a. This plane synovial joint assists in providing GH joint stability primarily in the superior plane or motion.
   b. This joint is commonly injured when blunt trauma occurs.
      i. These are very common in falls and sports injuries where the AC ligaments are torn and the clavicle is displaced superiorly.
3. The Sternoclavicular (SC) Joint:
   a. This saddle joint articulates with the medial end of the clavicle on the sternum.
   b. This joint is often overlooked in evaluation procedures, but contributes to shoulder range of motion.
4. The Scapulothoracic (ST) Joint:
   a. This functional joint is comprised of the scapula moving on the thorax.
   b. Scapular mobility is essential in attaining full shoulder range of motion.
   c. Scapular stability is essential for minimizing stress of the weaker Rotator Cuff muscles, especially the Supraspinatus.
B. There is a balance in the movement of each of these four joints that must be maintained in order to prevent pathology, or effectively and efficiently rehabilitate the shoulder known as the Scapulothoracic-Glenohumeral Rhythm:
   1. For shoulder Abduction, the ST joint will contribute 60 degrees of motion and the GH joint will contribute 115 degrees of motion.
      a. The remaining 5 degrees of shoulder Abduction comes from the AC and SC joint contributions.
C. Shoulder strength imbalances in the major muscles that control the shoulder complex are as follows:
   1. Those that are typically too strong and/or tight include:

        a.   Pectoralis Major, Upper Trapezius, Deltoid, Biceps, Triceps, Infraspinatus.

    2.   Those that are typically too weak and/or loose include:

        a.   Serratus Anterior, Middle and Lower Trapezius, Rhomboid Major, Rhomboid Minor, Latissimus Dorsi, and Supraspinatus.

    3.   Those that are typically balanced include:

        a.   Pectoralis Minor, Levator Scapulae, Subclavius, Coracobrachialis, Teres Major, Teres Minor, Scapularis, Subscapularis.

    4.   The four muscles that make up the Rotator Cuff are:

        a.   Supraspinatus (which is most often torn).

        b.   Infraspinatus.

        c.   Teres Minor (which is most often imbalanced/ weak).

        d.   Subscapularis.

    5.   It is wise to review the anatomical origins, insertions, innervations, and motions in order to fully and appropriately apply the proven therapeutic exercise techniques listed in this chapter.

        a.   This information can be found in the Appendix.

  D.   Based on the premise of "proximal stability for distal mobility" there is a proven therapeutic exercise progression in shoulder rehabilitation:

    1.   First, the Trapezius, Serratus Anterior, Rhomboids, and Latissimus Dorsi muscles should be exercised.

    2.   The second group of muscles that should be rehabilitated is the Rotator Cuff muscles:

        a.   Supraspinatus, Infraspinatus, Teres Minor and Subscapularis.

    3.   Third, are the Deltoids, Pectoral Major and Minor, and Biceps muscles.

        a.   Because these muscles are generally larger and less likely injured or involved in shoulder pathologies, their inclusion in the research is scant.

III. **Rotator Cuff Reflex Mechanisms:** [11,21,22,23,34,40,47,64,71,90,102, 109,110,113,117,119,140,143,146]

  A.   Any shoulder diagnosis involving pain will automatically shut down or reduce the contractility of the Rotator Cuff muscles:

1. The result of this reflexive shut down causes the Subscapularis and Teres Minor to NOT effectively work in force couple with the Supraspinatus to pull the humeral head inferiorly during shoulder flexion and abduction.

2. When this occurs, the Supraspinatus muscle migrates more superiorly than normal and often impinges on the Subacromial arch.

B. In normal operation, the Supraspinatus has maximal activity at 100 degrees of abduction.

1. This is also the point where the Subscapularis and Teres Minor provide an inferior force couple that prevents the humeral head and Supraspinatus muscle from impinging on the Subacromial arch.

C. Avoiding Supraspinatus impingement:

1. The primary movements that induce Supraspinatus impingement are shoulder flexion and abduction from the 60 to 120 degree arc.

2. The key to avoiding Supraspinatus impingement in rehabilitation is to limit initial activity of resisted shoulder flexion and abduction to 90 degrees or less.

a. In severe cases of Supraspinatus impingement, the motions of shoulder flexion and abduction may need to be limited to 60 degrees or less.

3. Furthermore, it is important to voluntarily contract the "Short Rotator Mechanism" upon initiation of resisted shoulder flexion and abduction.

a. The "Short Rotator Mechanism" is the term used to describe the force couple of the Subscapularis and Teres Minor muscles which provide directional force inferiorly and some internal rotation.

b. When voluntarily contracted, these muscles prevent humeral head migration in the superior direction which will impinge the Supraspinatus muscle against the Subacromial arch.

D. With this information in mind, we will now take a look at specific diagnoses and proven therapeutic exercise techniques for the shoulder.

IV. **Shoulder Hypomobility Diagnoses and Proven Therapeutic Exercises:**[3,4,10,34,44,47,51,63,64,70,71,77,106,115,123,137]

A. Common shoulder hypomobility diagnoses:

1. Adhesive Capsulitis.
2. Arthritis (Osteoarthritis and Rheumatoid).
3. Post Surgical Rehab.
4. Post Fracture Rehab.
5. Subacromial or Subdeltoid Bursitis.
6. Synovitis.
7. Tendonitis.
8. Sprengel's Deformity.
9. Pain.
10. Muscle Atrophy/Weakness.

B. Last Minute Reminders:
1. Range of motion and strength deficits, or imbalances, are easily evaluated in the shoulder girdle by comparing the involved shoulder with the uninvolved shoulder.
2. Make SURE the Scapulothoracic-Glenohumeral Rhythm is nearly 1:2 in ratio.
   a. There are many times where the Glenohumeral joint is limited and the Scapulothoracic joint compensates, thus becoming weak and overstretched.
   b. This can be avoided by securing a gait belt or secure strap around the patient's chest keeping the scapula from excessive winging and thus becoming unbalanced and hypermobile.

C. Proven Therapeutic Exercises for shoulder hypomobility:

4-1 "Pendulum"

Do NOT hold your breath.
Stabilize your trunk with the uninvolved arm.
Dangle the involved arm.
Gently initiate side/side, forward/backward, and circles 10 to 30
   times by moving your trunk using the uninvolved arm and lower
   extremities.

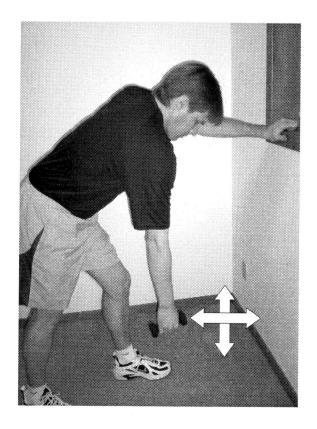

*The shoulder MUST be completely relaxed. (To test this, the clinician should apply a gentle force to the involved shoulder while dangling. The arm should naturally pendulate 2 to 3 times and stop.)

4-2 "Finger Ladder" or "Wall Climbs"

Do NOT hold your breath.
Slowly walk up the wall with your fingers.
Face the wall for flexion and turn 90 degrees for abduction.

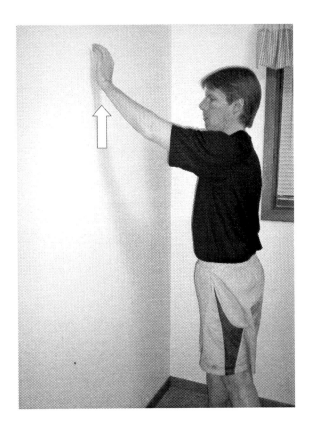

Hold at the top for 10 to 15 seconds, then walk down the wall slowly with your fingers.
Relax and repeat up to 25 times.

4-3 "4 Way Shoulder Isometrics"

Do NOT hold your breath.
Gently set the shoulder blades and hold.
Firmly press against an immovable object in all 4 quadrant planes of
motion.

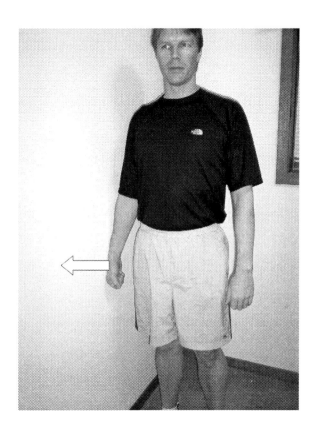

Hold 2 to 5 seconds.
Relax and repeat up to 25 times as tolerated.

*You may use oblique angles of isometric resistance if pure planar motion is not tolerated.

4-4 "Joint Mobilizations" These are primarily performed with "inferior" mobilization force in the movements of flexion and abduction. Minimal "anterior" planar pressure is applied to increase the movement of external rotation. Please refer to **Chapter 22** for specifics.

V. **Shoulder Hypermobility Diagnoses and Proven Therapeutic Exercises:**[3,4,10,34,44,47,51,63,64,70,71,77,106,115,123,137]
    A.   Common shoulder hypermobility diagnoses:
        1.   Muscle Strains.
        2.   Ligament Sprains.
        3.   Joint Dislocations.
        4.   Anatomical Deficiencies.
        5.   Cartilage/Meniscus Tears.
        6.   Pain.
        7.   Muscle Atrophy/Weakness.
    B.   Proven Therapeutic Exercises for shoulder hypermobility:

LEVEL 1 SHOULDER HYPERMOBILITY EXERCISES

4-5 "Shoulder Squeeze"

Do not hold your breath.
Press/retract your shoulder blades together

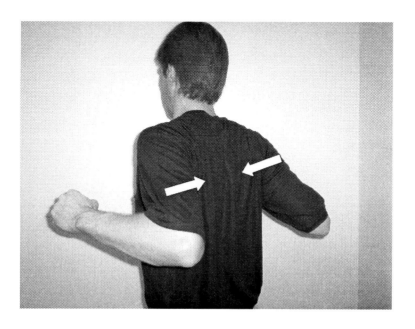

Hold >10 seconds as tolerated.
Relax and repeat 20 to 30 times as tolerated.

4-6 "Scapular Protraction"

Do not hold your breath.
Lay supine.
Keep your elbows extended at all times.
Protract or round out the shoulder blades as you push toward the
ceiling.

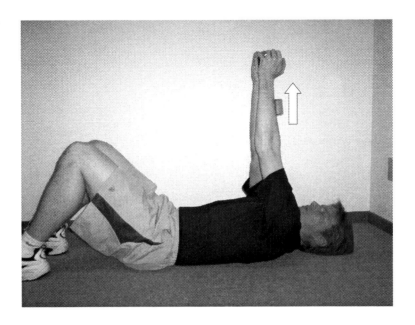

Hold 2 to 5 seconds.
Relax and repeat up to 25 times as tolerated.

*May use resistance bands or dumbbell weights to increase resistance.

4-7 "Lat Pulldowns"

Do NOT hold your breath.
Grasp a resistance band at shoulder height.
Pull downward and finish with your hands at hip level.

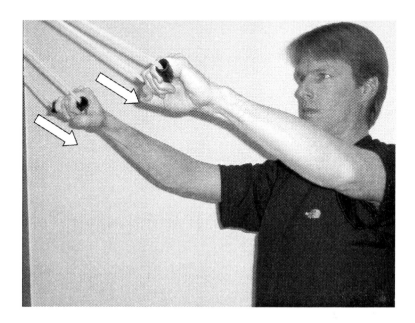

Hold 2 to 5 seconds.
Relax and repeat up to 25 times as tolerated.

*It is NOT recommended to start this exercise above the level of the shoulder, (i.e., 90 degrees) until the end stages of hypermobility.
*Do not progress to Level 2 unless symptoms are minimal.

Proven Therapeutic Exercise Techniques

LEVEL 2 SHOULDER HYPERMOBILITY EXERCISES

4-8 "Scaption in External Rotation"

Do not hold your breath.
Perform the shoulder squeeze and hold the position.
Keep elbows in contact with the abduction pillow.
Pull resistance band apart.

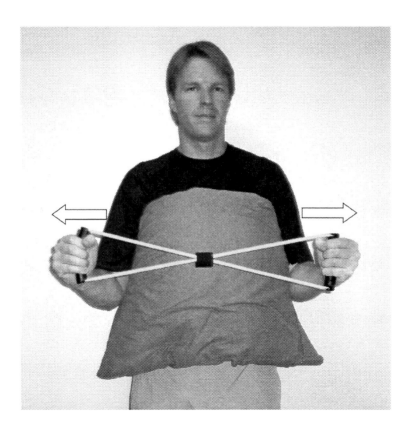

Hold 2 to 5 seconds as tolerated.
Relax and repeat up to 25 times as tolerated.

4-9 "Rowing"

Do NOT hold your breath.
Start from an extended arm position.
Pull backward using the shoulder blades first, then the arms.
*Do NOT allow your wrists back beyond the vertical plane of the hip

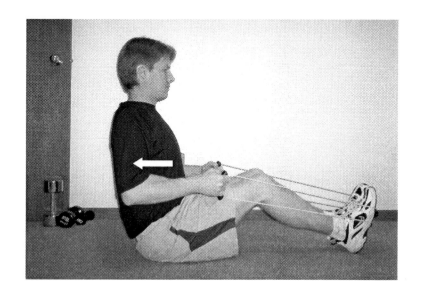

Hold 2 to 5 seconds.
Relax and repeat up to 25 times as tolerated.

4-10 "Push Up With A Plus"

Do NOT hold your breath.
(May start on knees if unable to keep an extended trunk on the toes)
Push up and ROUND out the shoulders at the top.

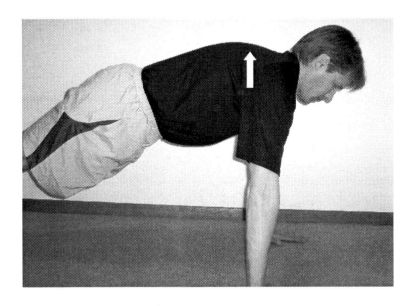

Hold 2 to 5 seconds.
Relax and repeat up to 25 times as tolerated.

4-11 "Press-Up"

Do not hold your breath.
Relax the back muscles and just use your arms.
Push your body up with your arms, leaving your pelvis flat on the floor.

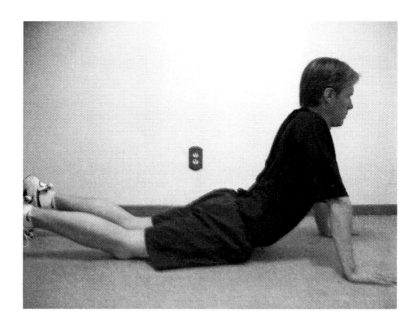

Hold 2 to 5 seconds.
Relax and repeat up to 25 times as tolerated.

*Do not progress to Level 3 unless symptoms are minimal.

LEVEL 3 SHOULDER HYPERMOBILITY EXERCISES

4-12 "Empty Can"

Do NOT hold your breath.

In the plane of the scapula, raise the involved arm with the thumb pointed upward.

At or before shoulder height, rotate the thumb downward as in emptying a can.

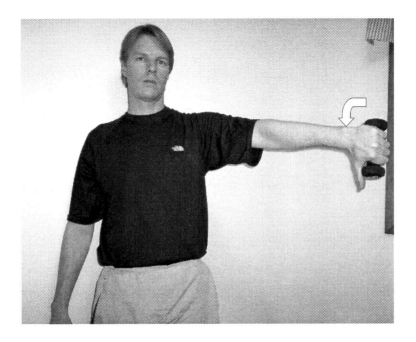

Hold 2 to 5 seconds.

Return thumb to upright position.

Relax and repeat up to 25 times as tolerated.

*It is NOT recommended to raise the hand/arm above the level of the Acromion (90 degrees).

*Dumbbell weights are the preferred method of resistance.

4-13 "Dumbbell Flys"

Do NOT hold your breath.

In the plane of the scapula, raise the involved arm with the thumb
pointed inward, (i.e., wrists horizontal, palms down).

Stop the movement at or below the height of the Acromion
(90 degrees).

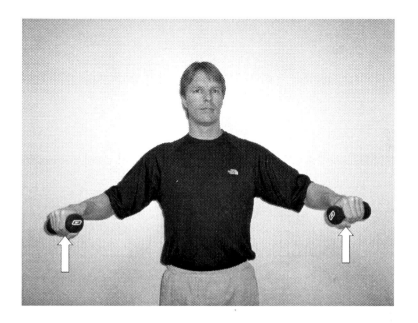

Hold 2 to 5 seconds.

Relax and repeat up to 25 times as tolerated.

*Dumbbell weights are the preferred method of resistance.

4-14 "Bicep Curls"

Do NOT hold your breath.

In the plane of the scapula, with the thumbs pointed outward, (i.e., wrists horizontal, palms up) bend the arm at the elbow pulling against resistance.

Keep the elbows in contact with the trunk pillow at ALL times.

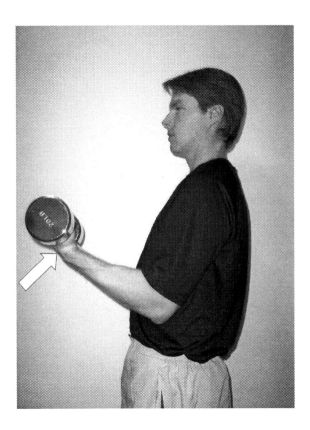

Hold 2 to 5 seconds.

Relax and repeat up to 25 times as tolerated.

*Dumbbell weights or resistance bands are the preferred methods of resistance.

4-15 "Triceps Extensions"

Do NOT hold your breath.
With the elbows in contact with the trunk pillow, point the thumbs inward and press down against the resistance.

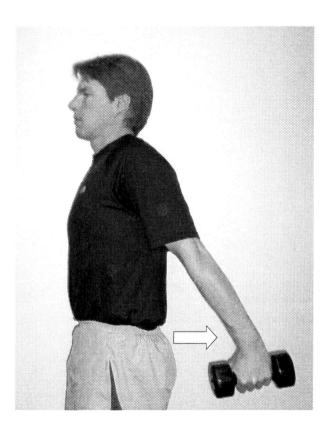

Hold 2 to 5 seconds.
Relax and repeat up to 25 times as tolerated.

*Dumbbell weights or resistance bands are the preferred method of resistance.

VI. **Shoulder Neurovascular Diagnoses and Proven Therapeutic Exercises:** [3,4,10,34,44,47,51,63,64,70,71,77,106,115,123,137]
    A. Common shoulder neurovascular diagnoses:
        1. Reflex Sympathetic Dystrophy.
        2. Shoulder-Hand Syndrome.

3.   Thoracic Outlet/Inlet Syndrome.
4.   Brachial Plexus Nerve Entrapment/Neuropathy.
B.   Proven Therapeutic Exercises for shoulder neurovascular conditions:

4-16 "High Corner Stretch"

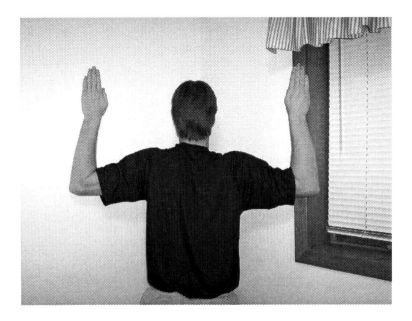

This stretch is performed by the patient placing one arm on each wall in a corner with the forearm (elbow to wrist) lying completely flat on the wall.
Perform 3 to 5 repetitions and hold the stretch 15 to 30 seconds each.

* It may also be performed while alternately extending the wrists and fingers while holding the stretch position.

4-17 "Neural Flossing"

Lay the patient supine (or sit upright) and side bend and rotate the head to one direction.
Provide simultaneous shoulder blade distraction to the side opposite of the head rotation.

Have the patient slowly extend the arm with the palm up.

Then have the patient slowly extend the wrist and fingers to maximum tolerance.

If pain and reproduction of symptoms occur upon the test, the brachial plexus extensibility is limited.

If the patient is unable to fully extend the wrist and fingers, brachial plexus extensibility is limited.

This test specifically isolates the median nerve with nerve roots C5-8.

Test left, and right arms separately.

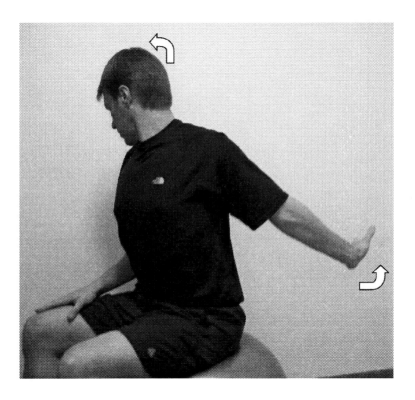

Hold stretch position as long as tolerated.

Flex and extend ("floss") the wrist/fingers 10 to 20 times as tolerated.

VII. Shoulder Post Fracture/Surgical Diagnoses and Proven Therapeutic Exercises:[3,4,10,13,34,44,47,51,63,64,70,71,77,106,115,123,137]

A. Common shoulder post fracture/surgical diagnoses:
    1. Shoulder Arthroscopy.
    2. Acromionectomy/Acromioplasty.
    3. Subacromial Decompression.
    4. Rotator Cuff/Muscle Repair.
    5. Total Shoulder Replacement.
    6. Cartilage Repair.
    7. Ligament Repair.
    8. Humeral/Clavicular/Scapular Fracture.
B. Proven Therapeutic Exercises for shoulder post fracture/surgical conditions by Brent Brotzman:
    1. It is IMPORTANT to note that these are a compilation of conservative rehabilitation measures for the aforementioned diagnoses.
        a. It is imperative that the treating clinician defer to the client's surgeon when treating.
    2. Collagen fibers begin to set up in 24 to 48 hours after surgery and other traumatic events.
        a. Therefore, it is imperative that the patients receive daily passive range of motion within pain tolerances of at least 10 repetitions for each involved joint and plane of motion.
    3. Phase 1 goals for weeks 0 to 6 are the gradual return to full range of motion and decreasing pain.
        a. This phase involves simple passive range of motion within pain tolerances of at least 10 repetitions for each involved joint and plane of motion.
        b. ABSOLUTE CONTRAINDICATED MOTIONS for Total Shoulder Replacements Anterior-Lateral surgical approach are:
            i.   NO shoulder external rotation.
            ii. NO shoulder abduction.
            iii. NO shoulder extension.
        c. A Kenny Howard sling or Shoulder Abduction pillow are often used after fracture/surgical intervention from 2 weeks to 6 weeks or more.

   d. Active/Resistive Exercises should be limited to the
       elbow, wrist and hand as tolerated.
   e. Scapular stabilization consisting of active shoul-
       der squeezes should also commence as soon as
       tolerated.
   f. The hypomobility exercises listed earlier in this
       chapter can be initiated. See figures 4-1 through 4-4.
   g. Pain relieving modalities are commonly used dur-
       ing this rehabilitation phase.
4. Phase 2 goals for weeks 7 to 12 are full, non-painful
   range of motion, and increasing strength and functional
   activities.
   a. Active Assisted range of motion (AAROM) is initi-
       ated in the early weeks of phase 2 as pain and
       symptoms tolerate.
   b. Active range of motion (AROM) and light resis-
       tance isotonic (RROM) are initiated in the later
       weeks of phase 2 as pain and symptoms tolerate.
   c. The hypermobility exercises listed earlier in this
       chapter can often be initiated. See figures 4-5
       through 4-15.
   d. Pain relieving modalities are used intermittently.
5. Phase 3 goals for weeks 13 to 21 are to maintain full and
   non-painful range of motion, improve speed and power,
   improve neuromuscular control, and gradually return to
   functional activities.
   a. Resisted Range of Motion (RROM) utilizing isoki-
       netic apparatus is often performed in this phase.
       i. Eccentric activities utilizing a medicine ball and
           rebounder/mini trampoline are also often per-
           formed in this phase.
   b. Functional closed chain (RROM) is also initiated in
       this phase as symptoms tolerate.
       i. A couple of the more efficacious exercises are
           listed here:

4-18 "Four Point Balance Board"

Do NOT hold your breath.
Stabilize yourself on your hands and knees.
Rock the balance board side to side and/or forward and backward with
    the arms in smooth fluid motion.

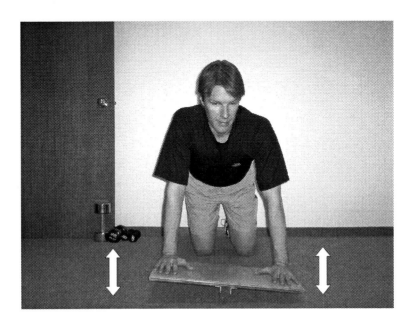

Repeat the right/left and/or forward/backward movements up to 50
    times as tolerated.

*BAPS (Balance And Proprioception System) boards may be used
also.

4-19 "Swiss Ball Arm Walking"

Do NOT hold your breath.
Stabilize yourself on the Swiss ball.
Walk yourself side to side and/or forward and backward with the arms
in smooth fluid motion.

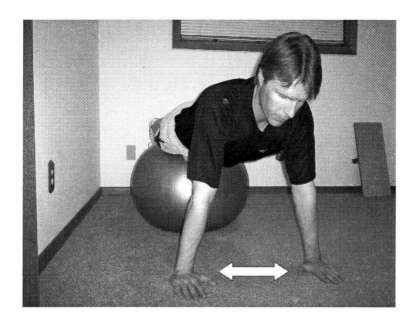

Repeat the left/right and/or forward/backward movements up to 50
times as tolerated.

6. Phase 4 is only initiated if return to sport or vocational
    activity require advanced rehabilitation.
    a. This phase normally continues 4 weeks beyond
        phase 3 rehabilitation and consists of sport specific
        activities and a variety of functional lifting and car-
        rying work hardening or conditioning.
7. Some advanced or rapid rehabilitation protocols for the
    less invasive surgical procedures such as Subacromial
    decompression and arthroscopy move the 4 phases of
    rehab from a 6 month rehab protocol to a 4 month time
    table with the same levels of activity as the standard re-
    habilitation protocols.

      a.   The following rapid rehabilitation time frames are listed below:

           i.   Phase 1 occurs in 0 to 2 weeks.

           ii.   Phase 2 occurs in 2 to 6 weeks.

           iii.   Phase 3 occurs in 6 to 12 weeks.

           iv.   Phase 4 occurs in 12 to 16 weeks.

8.   Please note that some physician protocols will even shorten the above time frames into a 12 week phase 1 through 4.

      a.   The key here is to remember that it takes a minimum of 6 weeks for tissue healing to occur in a healthy individual after the last trauma/micro-trauma has occurred.

      b.   Post-surgically speaking, there is micro-trauma that occurs at least until full range of motion is achieved which normally occurs in the first 6 weeks of rehab.

           i.   Therefore, tack on another 6 weeks and you get the justification for a 12 week rehabilitation plan.

      c.   Research is all over the board with the results of 3, 4 and 6 month rehabilitation protocols regardless of the joint being operated on.

           i.   Therefore, it is imperative that you use sound clinical judgment when treating and releasing your patients even when following the physician's protocol.

Chapter 5

ELBOW & FOREARM

I. **General Elbow and Forearm Considerations:**[20,34,47,51,63, 64,70,71,92,106,109,110,113, 115,123,137,141,146]

A. The elbow and forearm complex is highly susceptible to repetitive/cumulative trauma.

B. It is important to perform a complete musculoskeletal evaluation in order to determine the correct pathology and/or symptoms before proceeding with therapeutic exercise treatment.

C. One of the advantages with extremity evaluations is the fact that only one side is normally affected and the clinician may use the other side as a "normal" baseline.

1. Keep in mind that a 10 percent strength differential is considered normal for the dominant hand side.

a. For example, it would be considered normal in a right handed dominant individual to be 10 percent stronger on their dominant side.

D. The "Carrying Angle" is where the Trochlea articulates with the Radius and Ulna.

1. The "Carrying Angle" is 5 degrees of natural Valgus on elbow extension for men.

2. The "Carrying Angle" is 10 to 15 degrees of natural Valgus on elbow extension for women.

3. The "Carrying Angle" disappears with elbow flexion and forearm Pronation.

4. Knowledge of the normal amount of natural Valgus (i.e., "Carrying Angle") on elbow extension is important in order to insure normal stresses on the medial and lateral collateral ligaments during rehabilitation exercise.

D. Therapeutic exercise for balanced elbow and forearm rehabilitation progression:

1. The "PRICE" principle applies for all shoulder rehabilitation that involves inflammation and/or trauma.
   a. "P"rotection often means refraining from sport or activity.
      i. It may also involve a protection brace or Ace wrap.
   b. "R"est often means taking a break from activity.
      i. Keep in mind this excludes range of motion that requires 10 repetitions daily to maintain joint nutrition.
   c. "I"ce or cryotherapy will reduce pain and inflammation.
   d. "C"ompression will also reduce pain and inflammation.
      i. Ace compression wraps and neoprene braces/sleeves are commonly used for the elbow and forearm.
   e. "E"levation will prevent distal extremity edema and often involves laying supine or side lying on the uninvolved shoulder.
      i. Sitting and standing should be minimized.

II. **Elbow & Forearm Imbalances:**[20,34,47,51,63,64,70,71,92,106,109,110,113,115,123,137,141,146]

   A. Range of motion imbalances occur in the elbow and forearm complex which is made up of four anatomical joints:
   1. The Humeroradial (HR) Joint:
      a. This saddle joint creates the equal shares of range of motion for flexion, extension, supination and pronation for the forearm complex.
      b. This is the joint that is often dislocated as the Annular Ligament is easily compromised when stresses are applied in oblique angles.
         i. A common example of HR joint dislocation occurs in children when the parent grabs the child by the wrist and pulls them up, or the child drops to the floor.
         ii. This is affectionately referred to as "Nursemaid's Elbow" and can easily be reduced by applying a pronation rotational force to the forearm in combination with elbow flexion.

2. The Humeroulnar (HU) Joint:
   a. This hinge joint provides the majority of range of motion for elbow flexion and extension.
   b. This joint is commonly injured with repetitive pressure and trauma being applied to the Olecranon and often results in Olecranon Bursitis.
3. The Proximal Radioulnar Joint (PRU) Joint:
   a. This joint articulates with the proximal end of the Ulna and provides the majority of range of motion for Pronation and Supination.
4. The Distal Radioulnar Joint (DRU) Joint:
   a. This joint articulates with the distal end of the Ulna and provides minor, but essential range of motion for pronation and supination.
   b. DRU mobility is essential in attaining full forearm supination and pronation range of motion.
   c. This joint is often overlooked in evaluation procedures, but contributes to elbow supination and pronation range of motion.
B. There is a balance in the movement of each of these four joints that must be maintained in order to prevent pathology, or effectively and efficiently rehabilitate the elbow and forearm complex.
C. Elbow and forearm strength imbalances in the major muscles that control the elbow/forearm complex are as follows:
   1. Those that are typically too strong and/or tight include:
      a. Pronator Teres, Flexor Carpi Ulnaris and Flexor Carpi Radialis.
   2. Those that are typically too weak and/or loose include:
      a. Supinator, Extensor Carpi Ulnaris and Extensor Carpi Radialis.
   3. As we can see, the actions of wrist Extension and forearm supination is generally weaker and/or looser than the actions of wrist Flexion and forearm pronation.
   4. It is wise to review the anatomical origins, insertions, innervations, and motions in order to fully and appropriately apply the proven therapeutic exercise techniques listed in this chapter.
      a. This information can be found in the Appendix.

D. Based on the premise of "stretching before strengthening" there is a proven therapeutic exercise progression in elbow and forearm rehabilitation:
   1. First, stretches are to be applied to the forearm pronators and flexor muscles.
   2. Second, strengthening exercises should be applied to the forearm supinators and extensor muscles.
      a. Great care must be taken when exercising the elbow and forearm muscles as to reduce the likelihood of repetitive trauma or tendonitis.
      b. These muscles are generally smaller and more likely to be injured or involved in elbow and forearm pathologies.
E. With this information in mind, we will now take a look at specific diagnoses and proven therapeutic exercise techniques for the elbow and forearm complex.

IV. **Elbow and Forearm Hypomobility Diagnoses and Proven Therapeutic Exercises:** [3,4,10,34,44,47,51,63,64,70, 71,77,106,115,123,137]

A. Common elbow and forearm hypomobility diagnoses:
   1. Adhesive Capsulitis.
   2. Arthritis (Osteoarthritis and Rheumatoid).
   3. Post Surgical Rehab.
   4. Post Fracture Rehab.
   5. Olecranon Bursitis.
   6. Synovitis.
   7. Tendonitis.
   8. Lateral Epicondylitis (Tennis Elbow).
   9. Medial Epicondylitis (Golfer's Elbow).
   10. Pain.
   11. Muscle Atrophy/Weakness.
B. Last Minute Reminders:
   1. Range of motion and strength deficits or imbalances, are easily evaluated in the elbow and forearm complex by comparing the involved elbow/forearm with the uninvolved side.
   2. Remember to keep the "Carrying Angle" in mind when applying exercises as to reduce the likelihood of unnecessary ligament stresses.
C. Proven Therapeutic Exercises for elbow and forearm hypomobility:

5-1 "Dumbbell Supination Stretch"

Do NOT hold your breath.
With a dumbbell weight in the involved hand, stabilize the forearm and allow the hand to be off the edge of a plinth or table.
Slowly supinated the forearm and allow gravity and the weight to stretch the forearm.

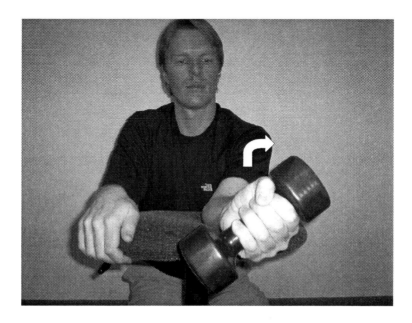

Allow the stretch 15 to 30 seconds.
Repeat 3 to 5 times as tolerated.

5-2 "Dumbbell Pronation Stretch"

Do NOT hold your breath.

With a dumbbell weight in the involved hand, stabilize the forearm and allow the hand to be off the edge of a plinth or table.

Slowly pronate the forearm and allow gravity and the weight to stretch the forearm.

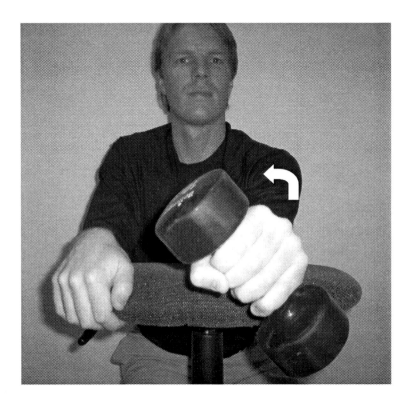

Allow the stretch 15 to 30 seconds.

Repeat 3 to 5 times as tolerated.

V. **Elbow and Forearm Hypermobility Diagnoses and Proven Therapeutic Exercises:** [3,4,10,34,44,47,51,63,64,70,71,77,106, 115,123,137]

    A. Common elbow and forearm hypermobility diagnoses:

        1. Muscle Strains.

        2. Ligament Sprains.

        3. Joint Dislocations.

4. Anatomical Deficiencies.
5. Cartilage/Meniscus Tears.
6. Pain.
7. Muscle Atrophy/Weakness.
B. Proven Therapeutic Exercises for elbow and forearm hyper-mobility:

5-3 "Corkscrews"

Do not hold your breath.
Begin with the elbow extended forearm pronated, holding a dumbbell weight.
Bend your elbow and simultaneously supinated the forearm.

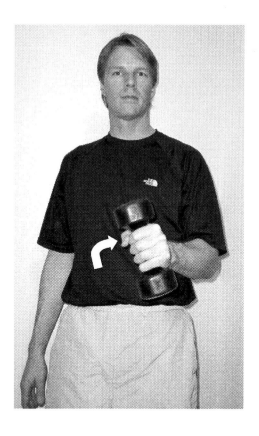

Hold 2 to 5 seconds.
Repeat 25 to 30 times as tolerated.

5-4 "Reverse Corkscrews"

Do not hold your breath.
Begin with the elbow extended forearm supinated, holding a dumbbell
  weight.
Bend your elbow and simultaneously pronate the forearm.

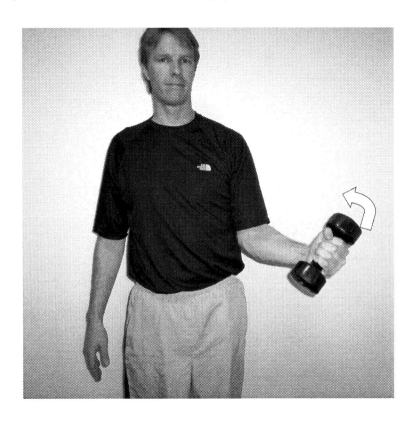

Hold 2 to 5 seconds.
Repeat 25 to 30 times as tolerated.

5-5 "Isolation Wrist Flexion"

Do not hold your breath.
Begin with the elbow stabilized on a table or plinth extended with the forearm supinated, holding a dumbbell weight.
Flex your wrist up.

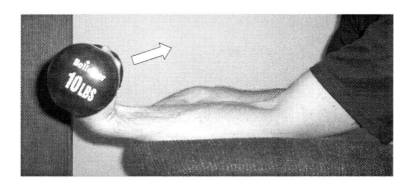

Hold 2 to 5 seconds.
Repeat 25 to 30 times as tolerated.

5-6 "Isolation Wrist Extension"

Do not hold your breath.
Begin with the elbow stabilized on a table or plinth extended with the forearm pronated, holding a dumbbell weight.
Dorsiflex/extend your wrist up.

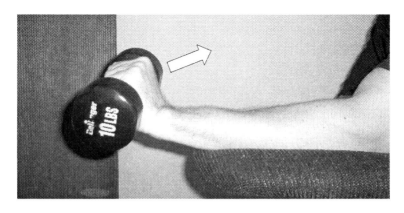

Hold 2 to 5 seconds.
Repeat 25 to 30 times as tolerated.

V.   **Elbow and Forearm Neurovascular Diagnoses and Proven Therapeutic Exercises:**[3,4,10,34,44,47,51,63,64,70,71,77,106,115,123,137]

   A.   Common elbow and forearm neurovascular diagnoses:
   1.   Reflex Sympathetic Dystrophy.
   2.   Shoulder-Hand Syndrome.
   3.   Thoracic Outlet/Inlet Syndrome.
   4.   Pronator Teres Syndrome.
   5.   Ulnar Neuritis.
   6.   Ulnar Entrapment.
   7.   Ulnar Neuropathy/Neuroma.
   B.   Proven Therapeutic Exercises for elbow and forearm neurovascular conditions:

5-7 "High Corner Stretch"

Do not hold your breath.
Place one arm flat on each wall in the corner of a room.
Lean into the wall until you feel a modest stretch in the chest and arms.
Dorsiflex/extend the wrists, hands and fingers to provide neural
   flossing.

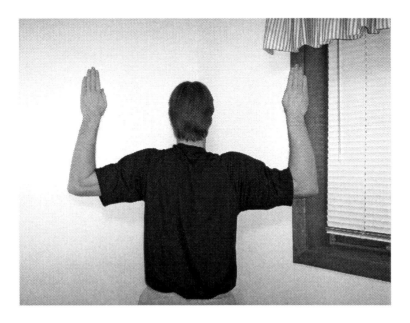

Hold the stretch 15 to 30 seconds as tolerated.
Relax and repeat 3 to 5 times as tolerated.

5-8 "Goose Neck Stretch"

Do not hold your breath.

Grasp your involved hand in a reverse goose neck position (wrist and fingers extended on the involved side).

Attempt to place the involved side fingers on the Deltoid muscle.

Slowly move the elbow up/down, in/out.

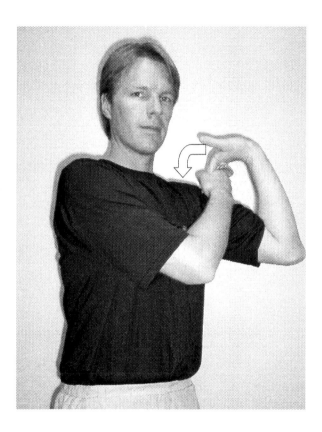

Hold the stretch position 15 to 30 seconds.

Repeat 3 to 5 times as tolerated.

VI. **Elbow and Forearm Post Fracture/Surgical Diagnoses and Proven Therapeutic Exercises:** [3,4,10,13,34,44,47,51,63,64,70,71,77,106,115,123,137]

    A.   Common elbow and forearm post fracture/surgical diagnoses:

        1.   Total Elbow Replacement (TER).

        2.   Flexor Tendon Repair.

        3.   Cartilage Repair.

        4.   Medial Collateral Ligament Repair.

        5.   Lateral Collateral Ligament Repair.

        6.   Radius/Ulna Fractures.

        7.   Ulnar Nerve Transposition.

B.   Proven Therapeutic Exercises for elbow and forearm post fracture/surgical conditions by Brent Brotzman:

        1.   It is IMPORTANT to note that these are a compilation of conservative rehabilitation measures for the afore-mentioned diagnoses.

           a.   It is imperative that the treating clinician defer to the client's surgeon when treating.

        2.   Collagen fibers begin to set up in 24 to 48 hours after surgery and other traumatic events.

           a.   Therefore, it is imperative that the patients receive daily passive range of motion within pain tolerances of at least 10 repetitions for each involved joint and plane of motion.

        3.   It is also IMPORTANT to note the rehabilitation time table is shorter for the elbow/forearm complex due to the more sturdy structure of the joints, as compared to the multi-axial shoulder joint.

        4.   Phase 1 goals for weeks 0 to 2 are the gradual return to full range of motion and decreasing pain.

           a.   This phase involves simple passive range of motion within pain tolerances of at least 10 repetitions for each involved joint and plane of motion.

           b.   A Kenny Howard sling and/or Pancake splint are often used after fracture/surgical intervention from 1 to 2 weeks normally.

           c.   Active/Resistive Exercises should be limited to the shoulder, wrist and hand as tolerated.

           d.   Scapular stabilization consisting of active shoulder squeezes and hand pumping exercises should also commence as soon as tolerated.

           e.   The hypomobility exercises listed earlier in this chapter can be initiated with very light or no weight. See figures 5-1 and 5-2.

           f.   Pain relieving modalities are commonly used during this rehabilitation phase.

5. Phase 2 goals for weeks 3 to 7 are full, non-painful range of motion, and increasing strength and functional activities.

   a. Active range of motion (AROM) and light resistance isotonic (RROM) are initiated in the later weeks of phase 2 as pain and symptoms tolerate.

   b. The hypermobility exercises listed earlier in this chapter can often be initiated. See figures 5-3 through 5-6.

   c. Pain relieving modalities are used intermittently.

6. Phase 3 goals for weeks 8 to 12 are to maintain full and non-painful range of motion, improve speed and power, improve neuromuscular control, and gradually return to functional activities.

   a. Resisted Range of Motion (RROM) utilizing resistance bands, dumbbell weights and other apparatus is often performed in this phase.

      i. Eccentric activities utilizing a medicine ball and rebounder/mini trampoline are also often performed in this phase.

   b. Functional exercises are also initiated in this phase as symptoms tolerate and generally consist of throwing activities.

7. Phase 4 is only initiated if return to sport or vocational activity requires advanced rehabilitation. This phase normally continues 4 weeks beyond phase 3 rehabilitation and consists of sport specific activities and a variety of functional lifting and carrying work hardening or conditioning.

   a. Keep in mind that athletes with throwing related injuries and surgical repairs such as medial collateral ligament reconstruction require nearly 7 to 8 months before throwing can occur at full speed.

8. Some advanced or rapid rehabilitation protocols for the less invasive surgical procedures such as arthroscopies move the 4 phases of rehab from a 4 month rehab protocol to a 2 month protocol with the same levels of activity as the standard rehabilitation protocols.

   a. This usually means the difference between surgical "Repair" and surgical "Reconstruction."

      b. The former "Repair" allows rapid rehabilitation protocols to be implemented in most cases.

      c. The following rapid rehabilitation time frames are listed below:

          i.   Phase 1 occurs in 0 to 1 weeks.

          ii.   Phase 2 occurs in 2 to 3 weeks.

          iii. Phase 3 occurs in 4 to 6 weeks.

          iv. Phase 4 occurs in 6 to 8 weeks.

9. Please note that some physician protocols will even shorten the above time frames.

      a. The key here is to remember that it takes a minimum of 6 weeks for tissue healing to occur in a healthy individual after the last trauma/micro-trauma has occurred.

      b. Post-surgically speaking, there is micro-trauma that occurs at least until full range of motion is achieved which normally occurs in the first 6 weeks of rehab.

          i.   Therefore, it is imperative that you use sound clinical judgment when treating and releasing your patients even when following the physician's protocol.

Chapter 6

WRIST & HAND

I. **General Wrist and Hand Considerations:**[20,34,47,49,51,60,63, 64,70,71,106,109,110,113,115,123,137,141,146]

   A. The wrist is the MOST complex system of joints in the body.
       1. Consequently the time tables for rehabilitation of the wrist, hand and fingers is substantially longer than that of the elbow and forearm complex.
   B. It is important to perform a complete musculoskeletal evaluation in order to determine the correct pathology and/or symptoms before proceeding with therapeutic exercise treatment.
   C. One of the advantages with extremity evaluations is the fact that only one side is normally affected and the clinician may use the other side as a "normal" baseline.
       1. Keep in mind that a 10 percent strength differential is considered normal for the dominant hand side.
           a. For example, it would be considered normal in a right handed dominant individual to be 10 percent stronger on their dominant side.
   D. Therapeutic exercise for balanced wrist and hand rehabilitation progression:
       1. The "PRICE" principle applies for all wrist and hand rehabilitation that involves inflammation and/or trauma.
           a. "P"rotection often means refraining from sport or activity.
               i. It may also involve a splint for the wrist and or fingers.
               ii. Common types of wrist/hand splints include: Functional Position Splint, Resting Pan Mitt Splint, Ulnar Gutter Wrist Splint, Dorsal Block-

ing Splint, Anti-Spasticity Ball Splint, Thumb Hole Wrist Cock-Up Splint, Radial Bar Wrist Cock-Up Splint, Dorsal Wrist Cock-Up Splint, Gauntlet Thumb Spica, Radial Gutter Wrist Spica, Wrist and Thumb Spica, and Dynamic Splints with Outriggers.

    b.   "R"est often means taking a break from activity.

        i.   Keep in mind this excludes range of motion that requires 10 repetitions daily to maintain joint nutrition.

    c.   "I"ce or cryotherapy will reduce pain and inflammation.

    d.   "C"ompression will also reduce pain and inflammation.

        i.   Ace bandages, Fingersocks and Coban compression wraps are commonly used for the wrist and hand.

    e.   "E"levation will prevent distal extremity edema and often involves laying supine or side lying on the uninvolved shoulder.

        i.   Sitting and standing should be minimized.

II. **Wrist and Hand Imbalances:**[20,34,47,49,51,60,63,64,70,71,106,109,110, 113,115,123,137, 141,146]

    A.   The "functional" position of the hand is important with regard to the discussion of wrist and hand imbalances. It is described as:

        1.   Slight wrist extension of 20 degrees.

        2.   Metacarpophalangeal flexion of 45 degrees.

        3.   Interphalangeal flexion of 30 degrees.

    B.   The "functional" position of the hand is the point at which there is perfect balance between the flexor and extensor muscles.

        1.   This position should be maintained as much as possible during rehabilitation of the wrist and hand in order to minimize inadvertent stresses on the joints.

    C.   Due to the fact that the wrist and hand flexor muscles are too strong and/or tight, as well as their superficial location, extensor tendon injuries occur 5 times more frequently.

        1.   Common wrist and hand extensor injuries include:

a. Mallet finger which affects the distal Interphalangeal joint and is treated with conservative immobilization for 6 to 8 weeks.

b. Boutonniere's deformity which affects the proximal Interphalangeal joint and is treated with conservative immobilization for 4 to 6 weeks.

c. Extensor Digitorum Communis tendon avulsion which affects the Metacarpophalangeal joint and is treated with conservative immobilization for 4 to 8 weeks.

D. Although less common, flexor tendon injuries also occur fairly commonly in the wrist and hand.

1. Common wrist and hand flexor injuries include:

a. Jersey finger in which the Flexor Digitorum Profundus tendon is avulsed normally occurring to the fourth (ring) finger and is treated nearly always with surgical intervention and immobilization for 4 to 8 weeks.

b. Trigger finger in which repetitive motion causes a thickening of the flexor tendon sheath and is normally treated conservatively with splinting and modalities.

c. Dupuytren's contracture in which the palmar fascia is contracted and there is a fixed flexion deformity of the Metacarpophalangeal and proximal Interphalangeal joints typically on the fourth and fifth fingers.

i. It is IMPORTANT to note that stretching makes Dupuytren's contractures worse and should NOT conform to the hypomobility exercises in this chapter.

E. With this information in mind, we will now take a look at specific diagnoses and proven therapeutic exercise techniques for the shoulder.

III. **Wrist/Hand Hypomobility Diagnoses and Proven Therapeutic Exercises:** [3,4,10,34,44,47,51,63,64,70,71,77,106,115,123,137]

A. Common wrist/hand hypomobility diagnoses:

1. Adhesions.

2. Arthritis (Osteoarthritis and Rheumatoid).

       3.   Post Surgical Rehab.

       4.   Post Fracture Rehab.

       5.   Synovitis.

       6.   Stenosing Tenosynovitis (Dequervain's Disease)

       7.   Tendonitis.

       8.   Ganglion Cyst.

       9.   Pain.

      10. Muscle Atrophy/Weakness.

B. Last Minute Reminders:

       1.   Range of motion and strength deficits, or imbalances, are easily evaluated in the wrist/hand by comparing the involved side with the uninvolved side.

C. Proven Therapeutic Exercises for wrist/hand hypomobility:

6-1 "Wrist Extension"

Place the involved wrist against a hard surface.
Press downward to bend the wrist until you feel a tolerable stretch.
Do NOT extend beyond a 90 degree angle.

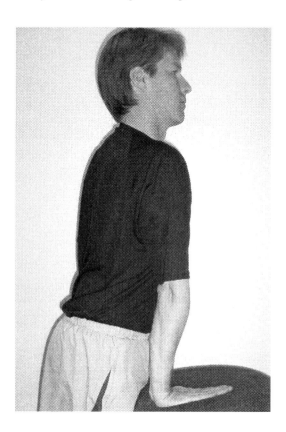

Hold 15 to 30 seconds.
Repeat 3 to 5 times as tolerated.

6-2 "Wrist Flexion"

Hold the involved wrist and bend it into flexion until you feel a tolerable stretch.

Do NOT extend beyond a 90 degree angle.

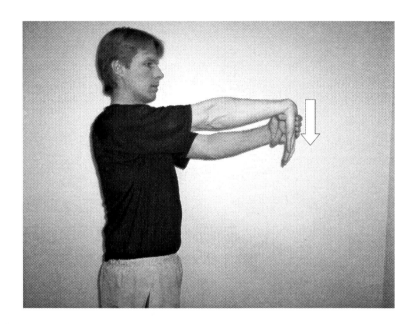

Hold 15 to 30 seconds.

Repeat 3 to 5 times as tolerated.

IV. **Wrist/Hand Hypermobility Diagnoses and Proven Therapeutic Exercises:**[3,4,10,34,44,47,51,63,64,70,71,77,106,115,123,137]

    A.   Common wrist/hand hypermobility diagnoses:

        1.   Muscle Strains.

        2.   Ligament Sprains.

        3.   Joint Dislocations.

        4.   Anatomical Deficiencies.

        5.   Cartilage/Meniscus Tears.

        6.   Pain.

        7.   Muscle Atrophy/Weakness.

    B.   Proven Therapeutic Exercises for wrist/hand hypermobility:

6-3 "Flexion Pinching"

Pinch a soft to medium firm material (putty or ball) between your index finger and thumb.
Hold 2 to 5 seconds.
Repeat the pinching procedure between your middle finger and thumb.
Hold 2 to 5 seconds.
Repeat the pinching procedure between your ring finger and thumb.
Hold 2 to 5 seconds.
Repeat the pinching procedure between your pinky finger and thumb.
Hold 2 to 5 seconds.

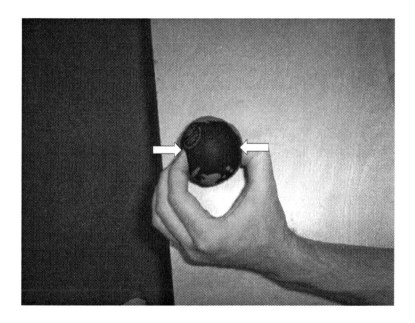

Repeat 15 to 20 times as tolerated.

6-4 "Adduction Pinching"

Pinch a soft to medium firm material (putty or ball) between your index
   finger and thumb.
Hold 2 to 5 seconds.
Repeat the pinching procedure between your index and middle fingers.
Hold 2 to 5 seconds.
Repeat the pinching procedure between your middle and ring fingers.
Hold 2 to 5 seconds.
Repeat the pinching procedure between your ring and pinky fingers.
Hold 2 to 5 seconds.

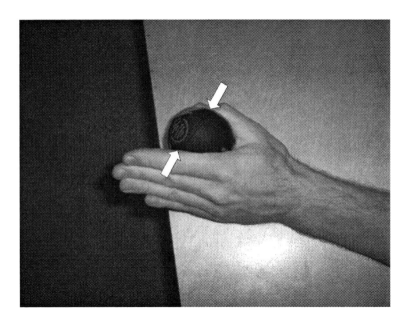

Repeat 15 to 20 times as tolerated.

6-5 "Finger Extension and Abduction"

Place a rubber band around the tips of all fingers and thumb.
Extend and abduct the fingers and thumb.

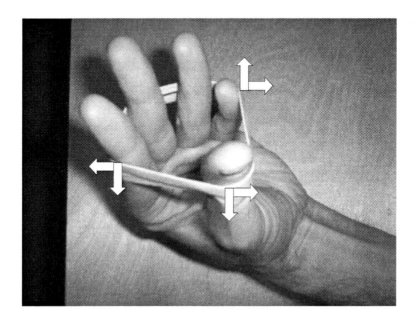

Hold 2 to 5 seconds.
Repeat 15 to 20 times as tolerated.

*May also be performed using resistance putty.

6-6 "Wrist Rolling"

Stabilize the forearms on a firm surface.

Place the hands palm down.

Roll the resistance weight up using the extensor musculature, then eccentrically lower the weight.

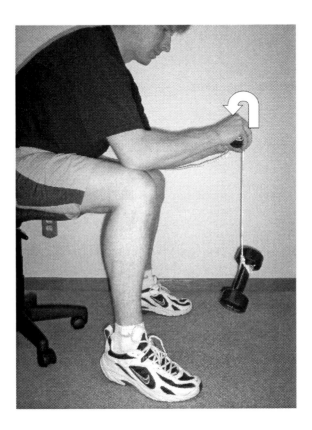

Repeat 15 to 20 times.

* Repeat this exercise with the palms facing up using the flexor musculature.

V. **Wrist/Hand Neurovascular Diagnoses and Proven Therapeutic Exercises:**[3,4,10,34,44,47,51,63,64,70,71,77,106,115,123,137]
    A. Common wrist/hand neurovascular diagnoses:
        1. Reflex Sympathetic Dystrophy.
        2. Shoulder-Hand Syndrome.
        3. Carpal Tunnel Syndrome.
        4. Cubital Tunnel Syndrome.

      5.   Guyon Canal Ulnar Nerve Compression/Cyclist's Compression.

B. Proven Therapeutic Exercises for wrist/hand neurovascular conditions:

      1.   Please note this sequential progression is to be performed from step one through step six 15 to 20 times as the patient tolerates per treatment.

      2.   Essentially this six step sequence provides minimally stressful nerve gliding for the median and ulnar nerves as well as ventral vasculature gliding/stretching.

      3.   The seventh exercise in this section is for isolating the radial nerve and dorsal vasculature for gliding/stretching.

6-7 "Step One"

Begin with a closed fist.
Wrist in "functional" position with fingers and thumb flexed.

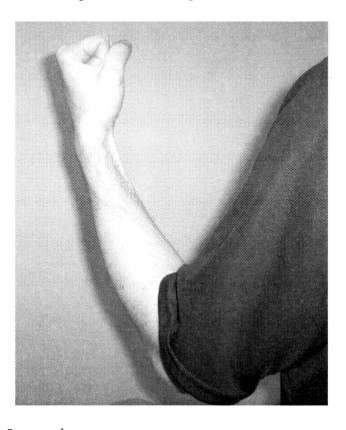

Hold 2 to 5 seconds.

Proven Therapeutic Exercise Techniques

6-8 "Step Two"

Keeping the wrist in a neutral position, extend the fingers and thumb.

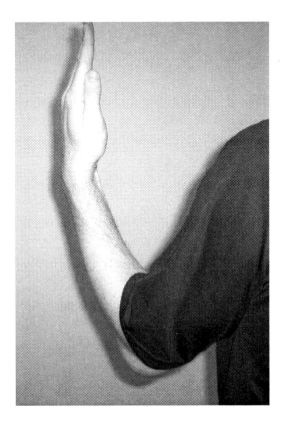

Hold 2 to 5 seconds.

6-9 "Step Three"

Keeping the thumb in line with the fingers, extend the wrist and fingers
   maximally.

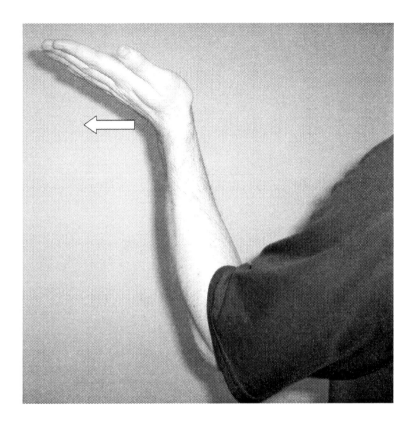

Hold 2 to 5 seconds.

6-10 "Step Four"

Holding the position in step three, extend the thumb maximally.

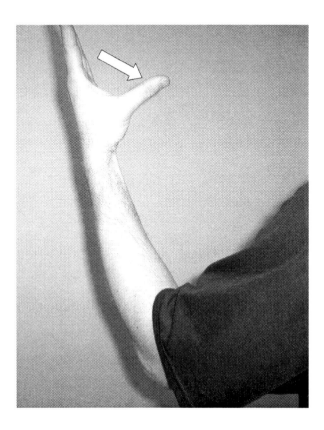

Hold 2 to 5 seconds.

6-11 "Step Five"

Holding the position in step four, now supinated the forearm.

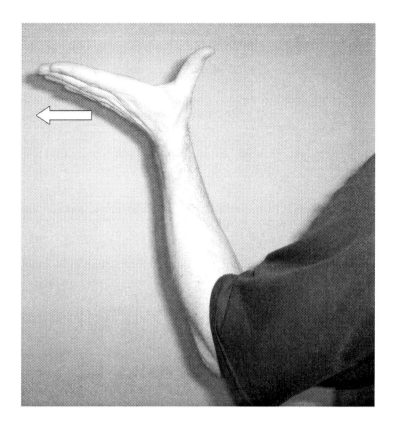

Hold 2 to 5 seconds.

Proven Therapeutic Exercise Techniques

6-12 "Step Six"

Holding the position in step five, now use the other hand to gently
stretch the thumb.

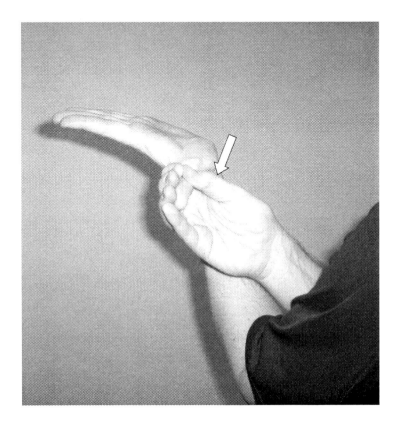

Hold 15 to 30 seconds.
Repeat at step one and sequence through 15 to 20 times as tolerated.

6-13 "Dorsal Nerve/Vasculature Stretch"

Extend the arm and elbow.
Actively flex the wrist and fingers maximally.
Reach back and try to touch all fingers and thumb together.

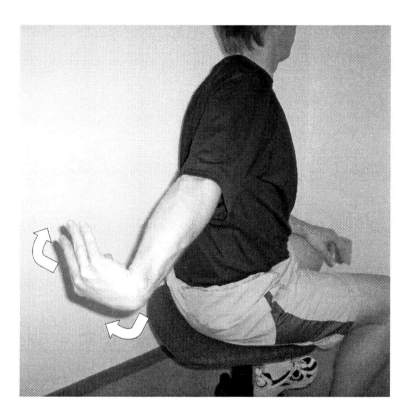

Hold 15 to 30 seconds.
Repeat 3 to 5 times as tolerated.

VI. **Wrist/Hand Post Fracture/Surgical Diagnoses and Proven Therapeutic Exercises:**[3,4,10,13,34,44,47,51,63,64,70,71,77,106,115,123,137]

    A.   Common wrist/hand post fracture/surgical diagnoses:
        1.   Wrist/Finger Arthroplasty.
        2.   Wrist/Finger Fracture.
        3.   Wrist/Finger Extensor Tendon Repair.
        4.   Wrist/Finger Flexor Tendon Repair.

        5.   Total Finger Replacement.

        6.   Cartilage Repair.

        7.   Ligament Repair.

B.   Proven Therapeutic Exercises for wrist post fracture/surgical conditions by Brent Brotzman:

    1.   It is IMPORTANT to note that these are a compilation of conservative rehabilitation measures for the afore-mentioned diagnoses.

       a.   It is imperative that the treating clinician defer to the client's surgeon when treating.

    2.   Collagen fibers begin to set up in 24 to 48 hours after surgery and other traumatic events.

       a.   Therefore, it is imperative that the patients receive daily passive range of motion within pain tolerances of at least 10 repetitions for each involved joint and plane of motion.

    3.   It is also IMPORTANT to note the rehabilitation time table is longer for the wrist/hand complex due to the more mobile structure of the joints, as compared to the elbow/forearm complex.

    4.   For most hand and wrist injuries/surgeries, (i.e., Flexor Tendon Repairs, Extensor Tendon Repairs, Fractures, Carpal Tunnel Surgery, Arthroplasty) the following guidelines exist but keep in mind each physician may alter these guidelines slightly.

    5.   Phase 1 goals for weeks 0 to 2 are the gradual return to partial range of motion and decreasing pain and swelling.

       a.   This phase involves simple passive range of motion within pain tolerances of at least 10 repetitions for each involved joint and plane of motion.

       b.   A Dorsal Blocking Splint for Flexor tendon repairs keep the distal and proximal Interphalangeal joints fully extended.

       c.   A Dynamic Cock-Up Splint with Outriggers is often used for Extensor tendon repairs to keep the fingers from forcefully flexing and avulsing the surgical reattachment.

          i.   Splints are often used for 2 to 6 weeks or more outside of treatment intervention.

      d.   Active/Resistive Exercises should be limited to the elbow and shoulder as tolerated.

      e.   Edema management using Coban or finger sock compression garments.

      f.   Initiate PROM within tolerable limits is initiated under skilled attention.

6.   Phase 2 goals for weeks 2 to 4 post injury/surgery include continued increase in range of motion and decrease in pain and swelling:

      a.   Sutures are removed.

      b.   Scar management treatment may begin.

      c.   Modalities like paraffin, whirlpools, fluidotherapy may be used to aid in range of motion treatment tolerance.

      d.   The hypomobility exercises listed earlier in this chapter can be initiated. See figures 6-1 and 6-2 as well as including the neurovascular exercise sequence figures 6-7 through 6-17.

      e.   Pain relieving modalities are commonly used during this rehabilitation phase.

7.   Phase 3 goals for weeks 5 to 8 weeks after injury/surgery are full, non-painful range of motion, and increasing strength and functional activities.

      a.   Active Assisted range of motion (AAROM) is initiated in the early weeks of phase 2 as pain and symptoms tolerate.

      b.   Active range of motion (AROM) and light resistance isotonic (RROM) are initiated in the later weeks of phase 3 as pain and symptoms tolerate.

      c.   The hypermobility exercises listed earlier in this chapter can often be initiated. See figures 6-3 through 6-6.

      d.   Pain relieving modalities are used intermittently.

      e.   AROM may begin.

      f.   Electrical stimulation may begin to facilitate muscle contractions.

      g.   Splint usually worn at night only.

8.   Phase 4 goals for weeks 9 to 12 weeks after injury/surgery are to maintain full and non-painful range of motion, improve speed and power, improve neuro-

muscular control, and gradually return to functional activities.

    a. Resisted Range of Motion (RROM) is the hallmark of this phase of rehabilitation.

    b. Functional and return to sports/work activities including lifting activities are performed during this phase of rehabilitation.

    c. Eccentric activities utilizing a medicine ball and rebounder/mini trampoline are also often performed in this phase.

    d. Functional closed chain (RROM) is also initiated in this phase as symptoms tolerate.

9. Phase 5 is only initiated if return to sport or vocational activity require advanced rehabilitation.

    a. This phase normally continues 4 weeks beyond phase 4 rehabilitation and consists of sport specific activities and a variety of functional lifting and carrying work hardening or conditioning.

C. Some advanced or rapid rehabilitation protocols for the less invasive surgical procedures such as Carpal Tunnel Release and Surgical Tenolysis move the 5 phases of rehab from a 5 month rehab protocol to a 3 month protocol with the same levels of activity as the standard rehabilitation protocols.

    a. The following rapid rehabilitation time frames are listed below:

        i. Phase 1 occurs in 0 to 1 weeks.

        ii. Phase 2 occurs in 2 to 3 weeks.

        iii. Phase 3 occurs in 4 to 5 weeks.

        iv. Phase 4 occurs in 6 to 7 weeks.

        v. Phase 5 occurs in 8 to 12 weeks.

    b. The key here is to remember that it takes a minimum of 6 weeks for tissue healing to occur in a healthy individual after the last trauma/microtrauma has occurred.

    c. Post-surgically speaking, there is micro-trauma that occurs at least until full range of motion is achieved which normally occurs in the first 6 weeks of rehab.

        i. Therefore, tack on another 6 weeks and you

get the justification for a 12 week rehabilitation plan.

ii. Therefore, it is imperative that you use sound clinical judgment when treating and releasing your patients even when following the physician's protocol.

Part 3

LOWER EXTREMITY
PROVEN TECHNIQUES

Chapter 7

PROVEN THERAPEUTIC EXERCISE TECHNIQUES – LOWER EXTREMITY

I. **General Lower Extremity Exercise Contraindications:**[3,4,][34,44,47,51,63,64,70,71,77,106,115,123,137]

   A. Common contraindications to active or passive exercise includes, but is not limited to:[12,14,19,26]

      1. Increased Inflammation.

      2. Unstable Cardio-Vascular Problems.

      3. Severe Osteoporosis.

      4. Ischemia/Peripheral Vascular Disease (PVD).

      5. Severe Pain Lasting More Than 24 Hours.

      6. Positive (+) Homan's Test For Deep Vein Thrombosis.

      7. Bony Block.

      8. Infection.

      9. Fracture.

      10. Malignancy.

II. **General Lower Extremity Exercise Precautions/Red Flags:**[3,4,34,44,47,51,63,64,70,71,77,106,115,123,137]

   A. It is critical to follow physician protocols regarding post surgical and post fracture care with their patients.

   B. These protocols ALWAYS supercede independent treatment plans and serve to protect the treating clinician from tort or malpractice legal actions.

   C. Red Flags for possible visceral pathology (i.e., cancer) include but are not limited to:[25]

      1. Weight Fluctuations.

      2. Inability To Sleep.

      3. Medications Are Required To Sleep.

      4. Pain Becomes Worse With Walking.

      5. Recent Fever Or Infection.

   D. Other Precautions include:

      1. Delayed Onset Muscle Soreness (DOMS).

      2.   Overtraining/Overwork.

      3.   Severe Osteoporosis.

      4.   Degree of Ischemia/Peripheral Vascular Disease (PVD).

      5.   Steroid Use.

      6.   Age.

      7.   Avoiding Valsalva Maneuver.

III. **General Lower Extremity Exercise Indications:**[3,4,10,34,44,47,51,63,64,70,71,77,106,115,123,137]

   A.   Common Diagnosis:

      1.   Arthritis (Osteoarthritis and Rheumatoid Arthritis).

      2.   Degenerative Joint Disease (DJD).

      3.   Post Surgical Arthroscopy and Arthroplasty.

      4.   Reflex Sympathetic Dystrophy.

      5.   Piriformis Syndrome.

      6.   Sciatica.

      7.   Pain.

      8.   Weakness.

      9.   Muscle Spasms.

     10.   Muscle Strains.

     11.   Ligament Sprains.

     12.   Post Fracture Care.

     13.   Myositis.

     14.   Osteoporosis.

     15.   Tendonitis.

     16.   Ischial Bursitis.

     17.   Trochanteric Bursitis.

     18.   Pre-Patellar Bursitis.

     19.   Pes Anserine Bursitis.

     20.   Baker's Cysts (Popliteal Bursitis).

     21.   Haglan's Deformity.

     22.   Iliotibial Band Syndrome.

     23.   Meniscal Tears/Internal Derangement.

     24.   Meralgia Paresthetica.

     25.   Morton's Neuroma.

     26.   Tarsal Tunnel Syndrome.

     27.   Contusions.

     28.   Adhesive Capsulitis.

     29.   Slipped Capital Femoral Epiphysis.

     30.   Legg-Calve-Perthes Disease.

     31.   Myositis Ossificans.

IV. **General Lower Extremity Exercise Goals/Benefits:**[3,4,34,44,47,51,63,64,70,71,77,106,115,123,137]

    A.   Increased Strength.

    B.   Increased Range of Motion.

    C.   Increased Flexibility.

    D.   Increased Endurance.

    E.   Increased Coordination.

    F.   Increased Agility.

    G.   Increased Balance.

    H.   Increased Speed.

    I.   Increased Stability.

    J.   Increased Function.

    K.   Decreased Pain.

    L.   Decreased Muscle Spasms.

V. **Lower Extremity Research Contributors:**[11,21,22,84,88,135,146]

    A.   This section is largely based on the research works by George Davies, Tab Blackburn, Mike Voight, Jenny McConnell and Steven Tippet.

        1.   They are experts in upper extremity rehabilitation and former or current affiliates with the North American Sports Medicine Institute.

    B.   These renowned therapists introduced me to the concept of muscle imbalances back in 1993.

        1.   What I learned from their research is the fact that muscle imbalances can occur from front to back (anteriorly to posteriorly) or right to left.

    C.   Muscle imbalances can result from a myriad of different reasons:

        1.   Dominant versus non-dominant sides.

        2.   Pain.

        3.   Incorrect strengthening and stretching exercises.

    D.   We are all familiar with the weight lifter at the gym who continuously works on the Quadriceps, but who ignores the Hamstrings.

        1.   The result is a typical anterior muscle imbalance which causes excessive anterior Tibial translation and subsequent Anterior Cruciate Ligament sprains or tears.

    E.   Another extremely common thing I encounter is the improper techniques people use when lifting weights and performing exercises.

1. The number one thing I see as a problem in this area is the fact that people perform exercises too fast.
   a. This causes them to recruit ancillary muscles to complete the exercises.
2. The second thing I see as a problem in this area is the fact that people consistently tear up their Patello-Femoral joint by performing deep knee bends and/or Quadriceps strengthening beyond a 90 degree bend in knee flexion.
   a. Knee flexion beyond 90 degrees causes extreme stress on the Patellofemoral joint and often results in progressive Chondromalacia and subsequent pain.

F. Due to the complex nature of the lower extremity, each of the following chapters are divided into the following:
   1. Hypomobile Conditions and Proven Therapeutic Exercise Techniques.
   2. Hypermobile Conditions and Proven Therapeutic Exercise Techniques.
   3. Neurovascular Conditions and Proven Therapeutic Exercise Techniques.
   4. Post Fracture/Surgical Conditions and Proven Therapeutic Exercise Techniques.
      a. The proven therapeutic exercises in each division may be applicable in more than one area depending on the diagnosis.
         i. For example in the post fracture/surgical division, the hypomobile exercises are generally applicable in the early phase of rehabilitation.
         ii. Whereas, the hypermobile exercises are generally applicable in the later phases of post fracture/surgical rehabilitation.
      b. Therefore, it is imperative that the treating clinician review ALL of the Proven Therapeutic Exercises for each condition and fully evaluate the patient prior to initiating a custom rehabilitation program for a particular patient.

Chapter 8

HIP

I. **General Hip Considerations:**[3,4,33,34,37,38,47,51,63,64,70,71,80,99,106,113,115,123,135,137]

   A. The hip is the MOST stable joint in the body.
     1. It is heavily reinforced by large muscles and ligaments despite its ball and socket type of joint allowing tri-planar motion.
     2. The femur is the longest, strongest and heaviest bone in the body.
       a. Despite this fact, the angle of inclination where the femur articulates with the Acetabulum is commonly fractured in the elderly due to the amount of force concentrated in that specific area.
   B. It is important to perform a complete musculoskeletal evaluation in order to determine the correct pathology and/or symptoms before proceeding with therapeutic exercise treatment.
     1. Anteverted femurs occur when the "Angle of Torsion" of the femur is greater than 15 degrees in adults.
       a. This results in the patient presenting as "knock-kneed".
       b. It also predisposes the patient to Iliotibial Band Syndrome, Trochanteric Bursitis and/or related knee and ankle problems.
     2. Retroverted femurs occur when the "Angle of Torsion" of the femur is less than 15 degrees in adults.
       a. This results in the patient presenting as "bow-legged".
       b. It also predisposes the patient to Piriformis Syndrome, and/or related knee and ankle problems.

C. One of the advantages with extremity evaluations is the fact that only one side is normally affected and the clinician may use the other side as a "normal" baseline.
    1. Keep in mind that a 10 percent strength differential is considered normal for the dominant hand side.
        a. For example, it would be considered normal in a right handed dominant individual to be 10 percent stronger on their dominant side, even in the lower extremities.
D. Therapeutic exercise for balanced hip rehabilitation progression:
    1. The "PRICE" principle applies for all hip rehabilitation that involves inflammation and/or trauma.
        a. "P"rotection often means refraining from sport or activity.
            i. It may also involve a hip immobilization/abduction pillow.
        b. "R"est often means taking a break from activity.
            i. Keep in mind this excludes range of motion that requires 10 repetitions daily to maintain joint nutrition.
        c. "I"ce or cryotherapy will reduce pain and inflammation.
        d. "C"ompression will also reduce pain and inflammation.
            i. Ace compression wraps in the form of a hip spica wrap are commonly used for the hip.
        e. "E"levation will prevent distal extremity edema and often involves laying supine or side lying on the uninvolved hip.
            i. Sitting and standing should be minimized.
II. **Hip Imbalances:**[3,4,33,34,37,38,47,51,63,64,70,71,80,99,106,109,110,113,115,123,135,137]

A. Range of motion and strength imbalances in the major muscles that control the hip complex are as follows:
    1. Those that are typically too strong and/or tight include:
        a. The hip flexors:
            i. Iliopsoas and Rectus Femoris.
        b. The hip adductors:
            i. Adductor Longus and Adductor Magnus.

      c. The hip external rotators:
         i. Piriformis.
      d. The hip abductors:
         i. Tensor Fascia Latae.
    2. Those that are typically too weak and/or loose include:
      a. Sartorius, Semimembranosus, Semitendinosus, Biceps Femoris and Gracilis.
         i. The hamstring group is made up of the Semimembranosus, Semitendinosus and Biceps Femoris and often weak and tight as opposed to week and loose.

B. The Pes Anserine is a common site for bursitis and medial knee pain that is a convergence of three muscle tendons indicating three different planes of motion that are often unbalanced and may involve one or more of the following:
    1. Semitendinosus which provides primary hip extension.
    2. Gracilis which provides primary hip adduction.
    3. Sartorius which provides combination hip flexion and external rotation.

C. It is wise to review the anatomical origins, insertions, innervations, and motions in order to fully and appropriately apply the proven therapeutic exercise techniques listed in this chapter. This information can be found in the Appendix.

D. With this information in mind, we will now take a look at specific diagnoses and proven therapeutic exercise techniques for the hip.

III. **Hip Hypomobility Diagnoses and Proven Therapeutic Exercises:**[3,4,10,33,34,37,38,47,51,63,64,70,71,80,99,106,113,115,123,135,137]

A. Common hip hypomobility diagnoses:
    1. Adhesive Capsulitis.
    2. Arthritis (Osteoarthritis and Rheumatoid).
    3. Post Surgical Rehab.
    4. Post Fracture Rehab.
    5. Ischial, Pes Anserinus and Trochanteric Bursitis.
    6. Myositis.
    7. Tendonitis.
    8. Iliotibial Band Syndrome.
    9. Pain.
    10. Muscle Atrophy/Weakness.
    11. Muscle Spasms.

   12. Contusions.
   13. Slipped Capital Femoral Epiphysis.
   14. Legg-Calve-Perthes Disease.
   15. Myositis Ossificans.
  B. Last Minute Reminders:
   1. Range of motion and strength deficits, or imbalances, are easily evaluated in the hip by comparing the involved hip with the uninvolved hip.
  C. Proven Therapeutic Exercises for hip hypomobility:

8-1 "3 Way Stretch"

Do NOT hold your breath.

Sitting with the legs extended and spread apart.

Keep your back straight and lean toward the right foot and hold 15 to 30 seconds.

Then lean toward the left foot and hold 15 to 30 seconds.

Then lean toward the middle and hold 15 to 30 seconds.

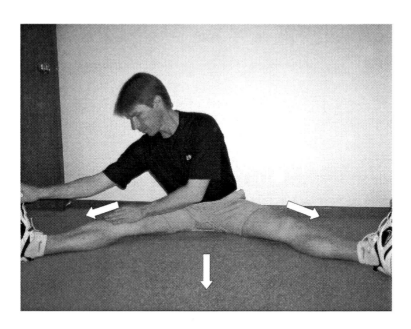

Relax and repeat 3 to 5 times as tolerated.

*You may dorsiflex the foot on stretching to elicit neural flossing.

8-2 "Piriformis Stretch"

Do not hold your breath.

Lay supine and cross the legs.

*Sitting upright and crossing the legs is an acceptable position substitute for those who cannot lay supine or who may have excess central obesity.

Pull the knee that is on top of the other up and across the body to the opposite shoulder.

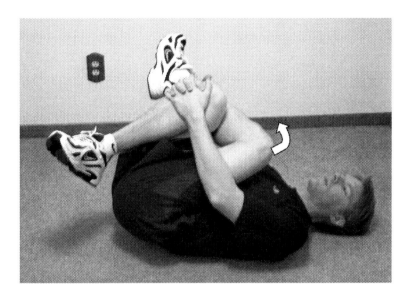

Hold 15 to 30 seconds as tolerated.

Relax and repeat 3 to 5 times as tolerated.

8-3 "Hip Flexor Stretch"

Do NOT hold your breath.
Gently push the heel toward the buttocks until tissue resistance is felt.

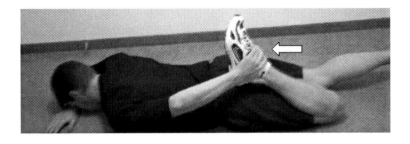

Hold 15 to 30 seconds.
Relax and repeat 3 to 5 times as tolerated.

8-4 "Iliotibial Band/Hip Abductor Stretch"

Do not hold your breath.
Keep the leg extended and stand approximately 8 inches from a wall.
Lean your buttocks toward the wall and hold the stretch position.
*You may need to vary the degree of hip flexion/extension in order to stretch the involved portion.

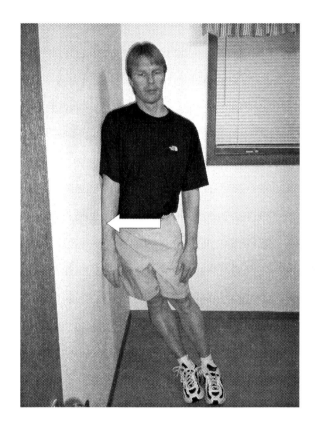

Hold 15 to 30 seconds.
Relax and repeat 3 to 5 times as tolerated.

IV. **Hip Hypermobility Diagnoses and Proven Therapeutic Exercises:** [3,4,10,33,34,37,38,47,51,63,64,70,71,80,99,106,113,115,123,135,137]

    A. Common hip hypermobility diagnoses:

        1. Muscle Strains.

        2. Ligament Sprains.

        3. Joint Dislocations.

      4.   Anatomical Deficiencies.
      5.   Pain.
      6.   Muscle Atrophy/Weakness.
  B. Proven Therapeutic Exercises for hip hypermobility:

8-5 "Bridging"

Do not hold your breath.
Squeeze your buttocks together and lift 5 to 7 inches, then lower.

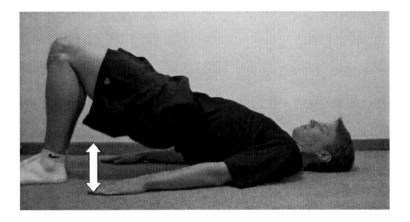

Hold 2 to 5 seconds.
Relax and repeat up to 25 times as tolerated.

*An alternate position to exercise these muscles is in the standing position and extending the leg behind the patient, if unable to tolerate the supine position.

8-6 "Straight Leg Raise"

Do not hold your breath.
Lay supine and bend the non-exercised leg at the knee.
Keep the involved leg straight and raise 5 to 7 inches as tolerated.

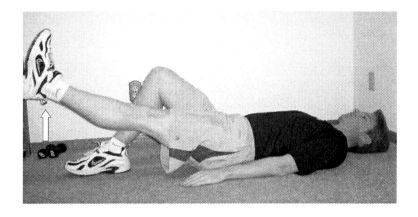

Hold 2 to 5 seconds.
Relax and repeat up to 25 times as tolerated.

*Alternate positioning for this exercise can be done standing.
*Resistance bands or cuff weights may also be used to increase the intensity of this exercise.

8-7 "Sidelying Hip Adduction"

Do NOT hold your breath.
Lying on your side, keep your leg extended and raise 3 to 5 inches.
The other leg may be behind the exercising leg, or crossed over it.

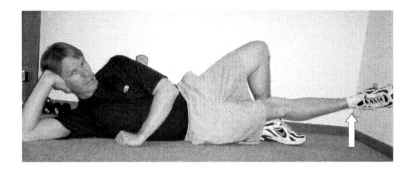

Hold 2 to 5 seconds.
Relax and repeat up to 25 times as tolerated.

*Alternate positioning for this exercise can be done standing.
*Resistance bands or cuff weights may also be used to increase the intensity of this exercise.

8-8 "Sidelying Hip Abduction"

Do NOT hold your breath.
Lying on your side, keep your leg extended and raise 5 to 7 inches.

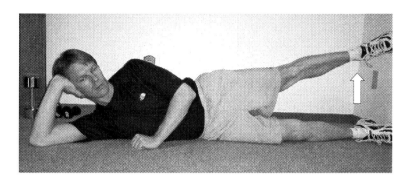

Hold 2 to 5 seconds.
Relax and repeat up to 25 times as tolerated.

*Alternate positioning for this exercise can be done standing.
*Resistance bands or cuff weights may also be used to increase the intensity of this exercise.

V. **Hip Neurovascular Diagnoses and Proven Therapeutic Exercises:** [3,4,33,34,37,38,47,51,63,64,70,71,80,99,106,113,115,123,135,137]
    A. Common hip neurovascular diagnoses:
        1. Reflex Sympathetic Dystrophy.
        2. Meralgia Paresthetica.
        3. Sciatica.
        4. Piriformis Syndrome.
    B. Proven Therapeutic Exercises for hip neurovascular conditions:

8-9 "LLTT–Lower Limb Tissue Tension Stretch"

Do not hold your breath.

Round out the spine (if no spinal pathology contraindicates this position).

Have the patient SLOWLY dorsiflex and plantarflex the foot 10 to 20 times as tolerated for neural flossing effects.

Pain or discomfort in the sciatic distribution along the hamstring is normal.

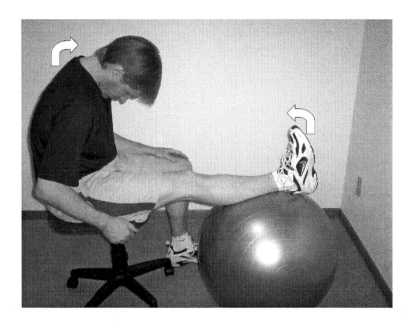

Hold 15 to 30 seconds each.

Relax and repeat 3 to 5 times as tolerated.

8-10 "Hip Flexor Stretch"

Do NOT hold your breath.
Gently push the heel toward the buttocks until tissue resistance is felt.
Maximally dorsiflex and plantarflex the foot 10 to 20 times as tolerated
for neural flossing effects.

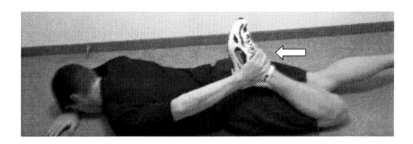

Hold 15 to 30 seconds.
Relax and repeat 3 to 5 times as tolerated.

*May vary degree of internal and external hip rotation during the
stretch to maximize the Lateral Femoral Cutaneous Nerve stretch for
maximal effectiveness in Meralgia Paresthetica.
*Ultrasound or Phonophoresis near the Anterior Superior Iliac Spine
(ASIS) is also efficacious for reducing Meralgia Paresthetica symptoms.

VII. **Hip Post Fracture/Surgical Diagnoses and Proven Therapeutic Exercises:** [3,4,10,13,33,34,37,38,47,51,63,64,70,71,80,99,106,113,115,123,135,137]

 A. Common hip post fracture/surgical diagnoses:
  1. Hip Arthroscopy.
  2. Total Hip Replacement (THR).
  3. Femoral Neck Fracture with Intramedullary Fixation.
  4. Femoral Shaft Fracture with Plate and Screw Fixation.
  5. Ligament Repair.
  6. Cartilage Repair.
 B. Proven Therapeutic Exercises for hip post fracture/surgical conditions by Brent Brotzman:
  1. It is IMPORTANT to note that these are a compilation of conservative rehabilitation measures for the afore-mentioned diagnoses.

    a.   It is imperative that the treating clinician defer to the client's surgeon when treating.

2.   Collagen fibers begin to set up in 24 to 48 hours after surgery and other traumatic events.

    a.   Therefore, it is imperative that the patients receive daily passive range of motion within pain tolerances of at least 10 repetitions for each involved joint and plane of motion.

3.   Phase 1 goals for weeks 0 to 6 are the gradual return to full range of motion and decreasing pain. This phase involves simple passive range of motion within pain tolerances of at least 10 repetitions for each involved joint and plane of motion.

    a.   A hip abduction pillow are often used after fracture/surgical intervention from 2 weeks to 6 weeks or more.

    b.   Active/Resistive Exercises should be limited to the knee and ankle as tolerated.

        i.   Ankle pumps should commence immediately and continuously in order to minimize the potential for deep vein thrombosis.

    c.   Functional activities of walking begin immediately with assistance and assistive devices.

        i.   Physician protocols dictate the amount of weight bearing that can be performed.

        ii.   I have worked with physicians who allow everything from toe touch to partial to weight bearing as tolerated after surgery.

    d.   Pain relieving modalities are commonly used during this rehabilitation phase.

    e.   CONTRAINDICATED motions following Total Hip Replacement include:

        i.   No hip flexion beyond 90 degrees.

        ii.   No hip adduction beyond neutral.

        iii.   No hip external rotation beyond neutral.

    f.   Ankle Pumps, Gluteal Squeezes, Short Arc Quads, and 4 Way Hip Isometrics should also commence as soon as tolerated:

8-11 "Ankle Pumps"

Do not hold your breath.
Maximally dorsiflex and plantarflex your foot.

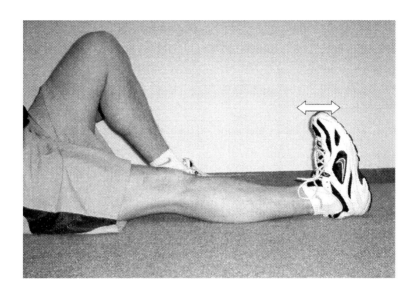

Hold 2 to 5 seconds.
Relax and repeat up to 25 times as tolerated.

8-12 "Gluteal Squeezes"

Do NOT hold your breath.
Squeeze your butt cheeks together.

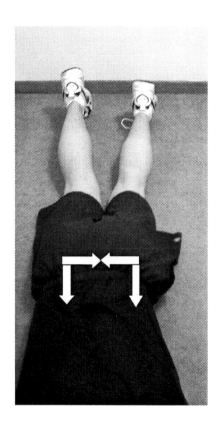

Hold 2 to 5 seconds.
Relax and repeat up to 25 times as tolerated.

8-13 "Short Arc Quads"

Do NOT hold your breath.
With a pillow/or rolled towel under the knee, push down into the pillow and extend the knee in a kick motion.

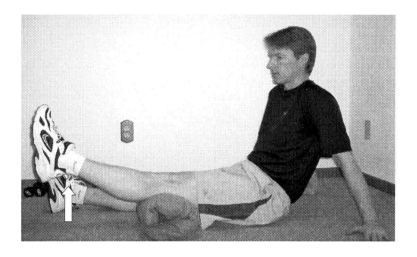

Hold 2 to 5 seconds.
Relax and repeat up to 25 times as tolerated.

*Cuff weights may also be used to increase the intensity of this exercise.

8-14 "4 Way Hip Isometrics"

Do NOT hold your breath.
Push in the four quadrant planes in neutral hip position against an immovable object.

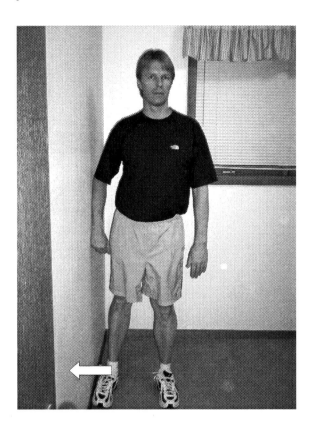

Hold 2 to 5 seconds.
Relax and repeat up to 25 times as tolerated.

*In the later weeks of phase one, cuff weights may also be used to increase the intensity of this exercise from isometric to isotonic in the standing position.

4. Phase 2 goals for weeks 7 to 12 are full, non-painful range of motion, and increasing strength and functional activities.

    a. Active Assisted range of motion (AAROM) is initiated in the early weeks of phase 2 as pain and symptoms tolerate.

    b. Active range of motion (AROM) and light resistance isotonic (RROM) are initiated in the later weeks of phase 2 as pain and symptoms tolerate.

    c. The hypermobility exercises listed earlier in this chapter can often be initiated. See figures 8-5 through 8-8.

    d. Pain relieving modalities are used intermittently.

    e. Functional activities such as walking are normally full weight bearing or weight bearing as tolerated.

        i. In some cases assistive devices can be discontinued in this phase.

5. Phase 3 goals for weeks 13 to 21 are to maintain full and non-painful range of motion, improve speed and power, improve neuromuscular control, and gradually return to higher level independent functional activities.

    a. Resisted Range of Motion (RROM) utilizing resistance bands and cuff weights are often performed in this phase.

        i. Balance activities utilizing a BAPS or Balance Board are also often performed in this phase.

    b. Functional closed chain (RROM) combination strengthening and balance activities are also initiated in this phase as symptoms tolerate. A couple of the more efficacious exercises are listed here:

8-15 "Side to Side Balance Board"

Do NOT hold your breath.
Stabilize yourself on an assistive device or with clinician support.
Rock the balance board side to side in a smooth fluid motion.

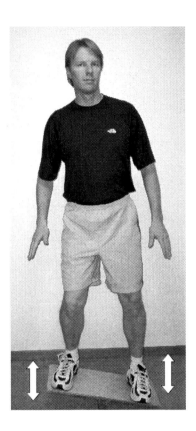

Repeat the right/left movements up to 50 times as tolerated.

*BAPS (Balance And Proprioreception System) boards may be used also to include circumduction movements.

8-16 "Forward to Back Balance Board"

Do NOT hold your breath.
Stabilize yourself on an assistive device or with clinician support.
Rock the balance board front to back in a smooth fluid motion.

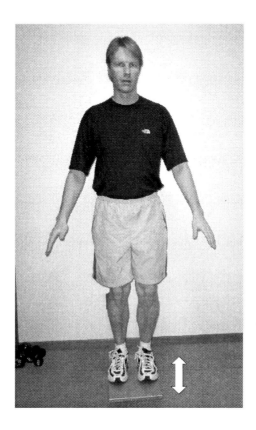

Repeat the forward/backward movements up to 50 times as tolerated.

*BAPS (Balance And Proprioreception System) boards may be used also to include circumduction movements.

6. Phase 4 is only initiated if return to sport or vocational activity require advanced rehabilitation.
   a. This phase normally continues 4 weeks beyond phase 3 rehabilitation and consists of sport specific activities and a variety of functional lifting and carrying work hardening or conditioning.
7. Some advanced or rapid rehabilitation protocols move the 4 phases of rehab from a 6 month rehab protocol to a 4 month time table with the same levels of activity as the standard rehabilitation protocols.
   a. The following rapid rehabilitation time frames are listed below:
      i. Phase 1 occurs in 0 to 2 weeks.
      ii. Phase 2 occurs in 2 to 6 weeks.
      iii. Phase 3 occurs in 6 to 12 weeks.
      iv. Phase 4 occurs in 12 to 16 weeks.
8. Please note that some physician protocols will even shorten the above time frames into a 12 week phase 1 through 4.
   a. The key here is to remember that it takes a minimum of 6 weeks for tissue healing to occur in a healthy individual after the last trauma/micro-trauma has occurred.
   b. Post-surgically speaking, there is micro-trauma that occurs at least until full range of motion is achieved which normally occurs in the first 6 weeks of rehab.
      i. Therefore, tack on another 6 weeks and you get the justification for a 12 week rehabilitation plan.
   c. Research is all over the board with the results of 3, 4 and 6 month rehabilitation protocols regardless of the joint being operated on.
      i. Therefore, it is imperative that you use sound clinical judgment when treating and releasing your patients even when following the physician's protocol.

Chapter 9

KNEE

I. **General Knee Considerations:** [3,4,9,15,16,21,25,28,33,34,47,51,63,64,70, 71,79,80,84,88,95,106,113,114,115,116,123,129,134,135,137,145,147]

    A.   The knee is the MOST often injured joint in the body.

        1.   Anterior Cruciate Ligament (ACL) is the MOST often injured ligament in the knee.

            a.   The mechanism of injury is usually hyperextension of the knee.

        2.   Medial Collateral Ligament (MCL) is the second most often injured ligament in the knee.

            a.   The mechanism of injury is usually a lateral to medial force in knee extension.

        3.   Lateral Collateral Ligament (LCL) is the third most often injured ligament in the knee.

            a.   The mechanism of injury is usually a medial to lateral force in knee extension.

        4.   Posterior Cruciate Ligament (PCL) is the fourth most often injured ligament in the knee.

            a.   The mechanism of injury is usually caused by extreme blunt force trauma from anterior to posterior commonly referred to as "Dashboard Knee" because of the high incidence in car accidents.

        5.   It is also important to note that nearly all ligament injuries in the knee have concomitant cartilage/meniscus injuries as well.

    B.   It is important to perform a complete musculoskeletal evaluation in order to determine the correct pathology and/or symptoms before proceeding with therapeutic exercise treatment.

    C.   One of the advantages with extremity evaluations is the fact that only one side is normally affected and the clinician may use the other side as a "normal" baseline.

      1.   Keep in mind that a 10 percent strength differential is considered normal for the dominant hand side.

          a.   For example, it would be considered normal in a right handed dominant individual to be 10 percent stronger on their dominant side.

   D. Anterior Cruciate Ligament (ACL) non-surgical management advocated by Shelbourne:

      1.   Non-surgical rehabilitation in combination with modified activity and bracing are effective in nearly one third of all ACL tears.

          a.   An important consideration for non-surgical management of ACL tears is the ability of the patient to develop and maintain strong hamstrings and calf muscles on the involved side.

              i.   A rule of thumb for hamstring to quadriceps strength follows a $\frac{2}{3}$ to 1 ratio.

          b.   Another important consideration for non-surgical management of ACL tears is the amount of anterior translation measured by an Arthrometer.

              i.   Non-surgical management of ACL tears is more likely to be successful if the anterior knee translation is less than 7 millimeters and no more than 2 millimeters more translation than the un-injured knee.

              ii.   KT-1000 and KT-2000 Arthrometers are standardized equipment utilized for these functions.

      2.   The remaining two thirds of all ACL tears require surgical intervention.

          a.   Common ACL repairs include:

              i.   Central $\frac{1}{3}$ Patellar tendon graft with bone plugs.

              ii.   Hamstring graft which has become more popular in recent years due to the strength and elasticity as well as decreased pain as compared to the central $\frac{1}{3}$ Patellar tendon graft.

             iii. Synthetic grafts.

          b.   Rehabilitation procedures are nearly identical for all 3 ACL reconstruction types.

   E. Therapeutic exercise for balanced knee rehabilitation progression:

1. The "PRICE" principle applies for all knee rehabilitation that involves inflammation and/or trauma.
   a. "P"rotection often means refraining from sport or activity.
      i. It may also involve a hinged or neoprene knee brace.
   b. "R"est often means taking a break from activity.
      i. Keep in mind this excludes range of motion that requires 10 repetitions daily to maintain joint nutrition.
   c. "I"ce or cryotherapy will reduce pain and inflammation.
   d. "C"ompression will also reduce pain and inflammation.
      i. Ace compression wraps and neoprene compression sleeves are commonly used for the knee.
   e. "E"levation will prevent distal extremity edema and often involves laying supine or side lying on the uninvolved leg.
      i. Sitting and standing should be minimized.

II. **Knee Imbalances:** [3,4,9,15,16,21,25,28,33,34,47,51,63,64,70,71,79,80,84,88,95,106,109,110,113,114,115,116,123,129,134,135,137,145,147]

   A. Mobility imbalances commonly occur in the patellofemoral joint of the knee:
      1. Patellofemoral pain is commonly seen in the athletic population due to strength imbalances in the Vastus Medialis and Vastus Lateralis of the Quadriceps muscle.
         a. That being said, the Vastus Lateralis commonly overpowers the Vastus Medialis causing lateral tracking of the Patella, pain and increased risk of dislocation.
      2. Lateral to medial patellofemoral joint mobilization and McConnell taping is often used as an adjunct to rehabilitation exercises and biofeedback specifically designed to strengthen the Vastus Medialis portion of the Quadriceps.
   B. ACL injuries are also predisposed due to the following conditions:
      1. Large "Q" angle which is the angle formed by a line from the Anterior Superior Iliac Spine to the mid

point of the patella connecting to a line to the Tibial tubercle.

    a.   Normal "Q" angles are 15 degrees.

    b.   Any "Q" angle more than 20 degrees predisposes the person to ACL injury which is more common in women than men.

2.   Weak hamstrings (less than ⅔ to 1 strength ratio between the hamstrings and quadriceps)

3.   Weak calf muscles.

III. **Knee Injury Reflex Mechanisms:**[3,4,9,15,16,21,25,28,33,34,47,51,63,64, 70,71,79,80,84,88,95,106,113,114,115,116,123,129,134,135,137,145,147]

A.   Any knee diagnosis involving pain will automatically shut down or reduce the contractility of the Vastus Medialis and medial Hamstring muscles:

1.   The result of this reflexive shut down causes the knee to become more unbalanced and unable to resist knee forces of anterior translation and normal Patellofemoral tracking.

2.   When this occurs, the Patella migrates more laterally than normal and often becomes dislocated.

3.   Furthermore, the reflexive shut down of the Semimembranosus and Semitendinosus portion of the Hamstring predisposes the ACL, MCL and Medial Meniscus to injury which is affectionately referred to as an "Unhappy Triad".

    a.   It is important to note that the Semimembranosus attaches to the medial aspect of the Tibiofemoral knee joint capsule as well as the Tibia and Medial Meniscus.

    b.   In contrast, the Semitendinosus is part of the Pes Anserine complex and contributes to medial stability of the knee by attaching to the medial condyle of the Tibia.

B.   In normal operation, the Vastus Medialis has maximal activity from 60 to 30 degrees arc of knee flexion motion.

1.   This is the arc of motion where biofeedback, electrical stimulation and exercise maximally strengthens the Vastus Medialis portion of the Quadriceps.

C.   Avoiding ACL stress during rehabilitation:

1. Closed chain exercise does NOT overly stress the ACL and is the reason much of knee rehabilitation is based on these exercises.
2. Open chain exercises does NOT stress the ACL from 100 to 45 degrees arc of knee flexion motion.

D. The knee joint also has specific roll to glide ratios in extension and flexion:
   1. Knee extension creates a roll to glide ratio of 1:2.
      a. The practicality of this ratio in knee rehabilitation is dictated by the structures involved.
      b. For example, if the ACL, PCL, Medial or Lateral Meniscus is injured you would want to maximize rolling and minimize gliding.
         i. Therefore, in these types of injury, you would want to exercise moving from greater knee flexion to lesser knee flexion angles.
   2. Knee flexion creates a roll to glide ratio of 1:4.
      a. The practicality of this ratio in knee rehabilitation is dictated by the structures involved.
      b. For example, if the knee joint is hypomobile you would want to maximize gliding and minimize rolling.
         i. Therefore, in these types of injury, you would want to exercise moving from lesser knee flexion to greater knee flexion angles.

E. With this information in mind, we will now take a look at specific diagnoses and proven therapeutic exercise techniques for the knee.

IV. **Knee Hypomobility Diagnoses and Proven Therapeutic Exercises:** [3,4,9,10,15,16,21,25,28,33,34,47,51,63,64,70,71,79,80,84,88,95,106,113,114,115,116,123,129,134,135,137,145,147]

A. Common knee hypomobility diagnoses:
   1. Adhesive Capsulitis.
   2. Arthritis (Osteoarthritis and Rheumatoid).
   3. Post Surgical Rehab.
   4. Post Fracture Rehab.
   5. Baker's Cysts/Popliteal, Prepatellar and Pes Anserine Bursitis.
   6. Synovitis.

       7.   Tendonitis.

       8.   Osgood Schlatter Disease.

       9.   Pain.

      10. Muscle Atrophy/Weakness.

      11. Osteochondritis Dissicans.

      12. Chondromalacia.

B. Last Minute Reminders:

      1.   Range of motion and strength deficits, or imbalances, are easily evaluated in the knee by comparing the involved knee with the uninvolved side.

      2.   To maximize Vastus Medialis contraction and minimize ACL impingement, keep in mind the arc of knee flexion that is concentrated for open and closed chain exercise is between 60 and 45 degrees.

C. Proven Therapeutic Exercises for knee hypomobility:

9-1 "Knee Flexion Hook Stretch"

Do NOT hold your breath.
Allow the involved knee to hang freely.
With the uninvolved knee, hook the involved ankle and press into
   greater flexion.

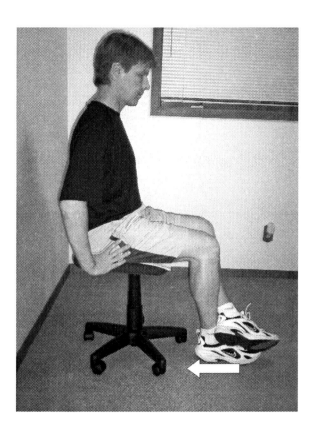

Hold the stretch 15 to 30 seconds.
Relax and repeat 3 to 5 times as tolerated.

*The knee MUST be completely relaxed. To test this, the clinician
should apply a gentle force to the involved knee while dangling. The
knee should naturally pendulate 2 to 3 times and stop.

9-2 "Knee Extension Stretch"

Do NOT hold your breath.

Prop the foot up on a rolled up towel or small bolster.

Place a small cuff weight on the anterior aspect of the knee and/or perform isometric knee extension exercises.

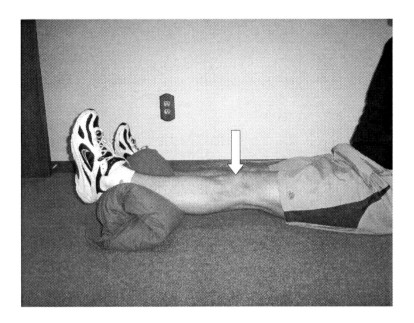

Hold for 15 to 30 seconds.

Relax and repeat 3 to 5 times as tolerated.

*Do not allow the knee to hyperextend for any reason.

9-3 "Multiple Angle Knee Isometrics"

Do NOT hold your breath.

At varying degrees of knee flexion and extension, gently set the quadriceps and hamstrings against an immovable object/clinician resistance.

Perform this every 10 to 15 degrees of knee flexion motion.

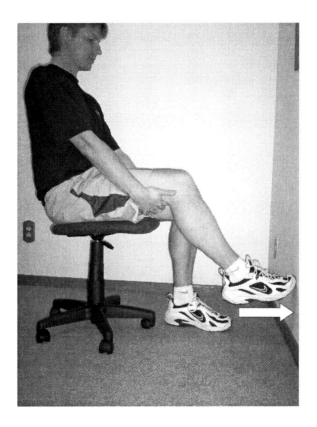

Hold 2 to 5 seconds.

Relax and repeat up to 25 times as tolerated.

*Remember to limit the angles of isometric contraction between 60 and 45 degrees of knee flexion in ACL diagnoses.

9-4 "Joint Mobilizations" These are primarily performed with "anterior" mobilization force to increase knee extension and "posterior" mobilization force to increase knee flexion. Please refer to **Chapter 23** for specifics.

V.　**Knee Hypermobility Diagnoses and Proven Therapeutic Exercises:**[3,4,9,10,15,16,21,25,28,33,34,47,51,63,64,70,71,79,80,84,88,95,106,113, 114,115,116,123,129,134,135,137,145,147]

　　A.　Common knee hypermobility diagnoses:
　　　　1.　Muscle Strains.
　　　　2.　Ligament Sprains.
　　　　3.　Joint Dislocations.
　　　　4.　Anatomical Deficiencies.
　　　　5.　Cartilage/Meniscus Tears.
　　　　6.　Pain.
　　　　7.　Muscle Atrophy/Weakness.
　　　　8.　Internal Derangement.
　　B.　Last Minute Reminders:
　　　　1.　Range of motion and strength deficits, or imbalances, are easily evaluated in the knee by comparing the involved side with the uninvolved knee.
　　　　2.　To maximize Vastus Medialis contraction and minimize ACL impingement, keep in mind the arc of knee flexion that is concentrated for open and closed chain exercise is between 60 and 45 degrees.
　　C.　Proven Therapeutic Exercises for knee hypermobility:

9-5 "Ankle Pumps"

Do not hold your breath.
Maximally dorsiflex and plantarflex your foot.

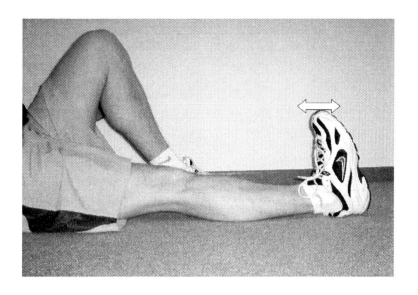

Hold 2 to 5 seconds.
Relax and repeat up to 25 times as tolerated.

9-6 "4 Way Straight Leg Raises"

Do not hold your breath.

Keep your knee fully extended and against gravity move the involved leg in the four quadrant planes of motion: Flexion, Extension, Abduction and Adduction.

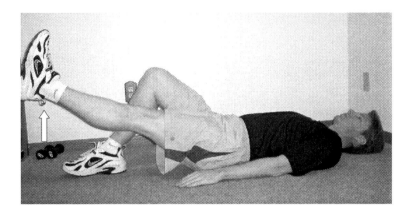

Hold each position 2 to 5 seconds as tolerated.

Relax and repeat 20 to 30 times as tolerated.

9-7 "Short Arc Quads"

Do not hold your breath.
With a pillow/or rolled towel under the knee, push down into the pillow and extend the knee in a kick motion.

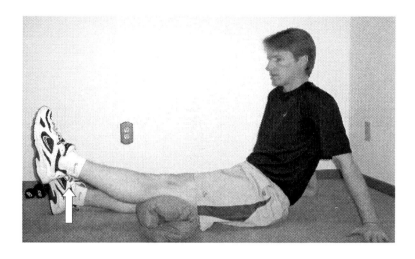

Hold 2 to 5 seconds.
Relax and repeat up to 25 times as tolerated.

*Cuff weights may also be used to increase the intensity of this exercise.
*Remember to limit the arc of motion in ACL injuries between 60 and
45 degrees of knee flexion.

9-8 "Heel Digs"

Do NOT hold your breath.

With the knee bent between 60 and 45 degrees of knee flexion, dig your heel into the floor/mat/plinth contracting the hamstrings.

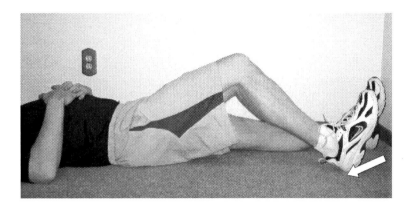

Hold 2 to 5 seconds.

Relax and repeat up to 25 times as tolerated.

*This may be performed open chain using resistance bands if not contraindicated by the knee diagnosis.

9-9 "Standing Heel Raises"

Do not hold your breath.
Keep your knees extended and raise up on your toes.
Use arm support for maintaining balance as necessary.

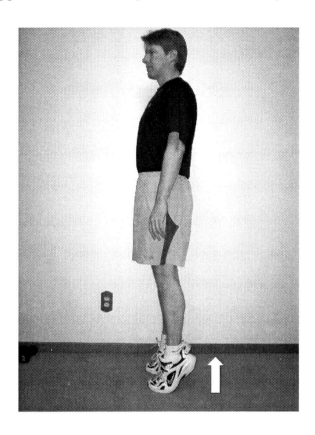

Hold for 2 to 5 seconds.
Relax and repeat up to 25 times as tolerated.

9-10 "Mini Wall Slides"

Do NOT hold your breath.
Lean up against a wall.
Slide down the wall about 2 to 4 inches.

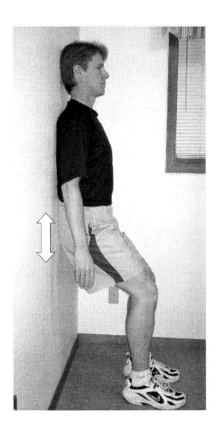

Hold for 2 to 5 seconds.
Then raise up and repeat up to 25 times as tolerated.

*NEVER squat down below a 60 degrees of knee flexion in ACL re-lated injuries.

9-11 "Step Ups"

Do NOT hold your breath.
Step up/down onto a stable platform anywhere from 2 to 8 inches high.

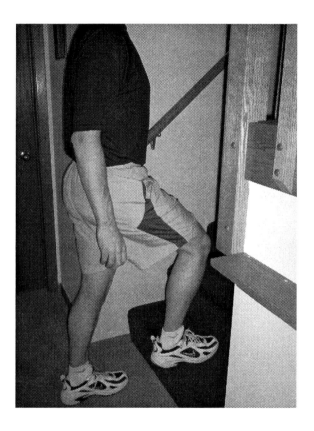

Hold 2 to 5 seconds.
Relax and repeat up to 25 times as tolerated.

*Make SURE the vertical plane is never compromised in step ups. In other words, the knee must NEVER go in front of the toes during this activity.

VII. **Knee Post Fracture/Surgical Diagnoses and Proven Therapeutic Exercises:** [3,4,9,10,13,15,16,21,25,28,33,34,47,51,63,64,70,71,79,80,84,88,95,106,113,114,115,116,123,129,134,135,137,145,147]

A. Common knee post fracture/surgical diagnoses:
   1. Knee Arthroscopy.
   2. Total Knee Replacement.
   3. Ligament Reconstruction (ACL, MCL, LCL, PCL).
   4. Ligament Stapling.
   5. Quadriceps/Hamstring Muscle Repair.
   6. Cartilage Repair.
   7. Femoral/Tibial/Fibular Fracture.

B. Proven Therapeutic Exercises for knee post fracture/surgical conditions by Brent Brotzman:
   1. It is IMPORTANT to note that these are a compilation of conservative rehabilitation measures for the afore-mentioned diagnoses.
      a. It is imperative that the treating clinician defer to the client's surgeon when treating.
   2. Collagen fibers begin to set up in 24 to 48 hours after surgery and other traumatic events.
      a. Therefore, it is imperative that the patients receive daily passive range of motion within pain tolerances of at least 10 repetitions for each involved joint and plane of motion.
   3. Phase 1 goals for weeks 0 to 6 are the gradual return to full range of motion and decreasing pain. This phase involves simple passive range of motion within pain tolerances of at least 10 repetitions for each involved joint and plane of motion.
      a. Continuous Passive Motion (CPM) machines are nearly always used immediately after knee surgery and provide daily PROM for the first week or two post-operatively.
      b. A hinged or neoprene knee brace is often used after fracture/surgical intervention from 2 weeks to 6 weeks or more.
      c. Active/Resistive Exercises should be initially limited to the ankle and hip as tolerated.

    d. The hypomobility exercises listed earlier in this chapter can be initiated in the early weeks of phase 1. See figures 9-1 through 9-4.

    e. The hypermobility exercises listed earlier in this chapter can be initiated in the later weeks of phase 1. See figures 9-5 through 9-8.

    f. Pain relieving modalities are commonly used during this rehabilitation phase.

4. Phase 2 goals for weeks 7 to 10 are full, non-painful range of motion, and increasing strength and functional activities.

    a. Active range of motion (AROM) and light resistance isotonic (RROM) are initiated in the later weeks of phase 2 as pain and symptoms tolerate.

    b. The hypermobility exercises listed earlier in this chapter can often be initiated. See figures 9-9 through 9-11.

    c. Pain relieving modalities are used intermittently.

5. Phase 3 goals for weeks 11 to 14 are to maintain full and non-painful range of motion, improve speed and power, improve neuromuscular control, and gradually return to functional activities.

    a. Resisted Range of Motion (RROM) utilizing isokinetic apparatus is often performed in this phase.

        i. Normally, isokinetic knee flexion and extension exercises begin with high speeds to reduce the torque and likelihood of injury.

        ii. In ACL rehabilitation, the Johnson Anti-Sheer device is required to reduce the anterior translation of the knee in isokinetic exercises.

    b. Functional closed chain (RROM) is also initiated in this phase as symptoms tolerate. A couple of the more efficacious exercises are listed here:

9-12 "Theraband Resisted Lateral Movement"

Do NOT hold your breath.
Perform and maintain slight knee flexion.
Stretch the theraband and begin to move side to side.

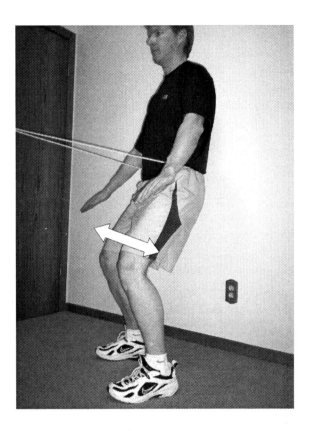

Repeat the right/left movements up to 50 times as tolerated.

*Remember to NEVER break the vertical plane of allowing your knee to extend beyond the toes.

9-13 "Theraband Resisted Forward/Backward Movement"

Do NOT hold your breath.
Perform and maintain slight knee flexion.
Stretch the theraband and begin to move forward and back.

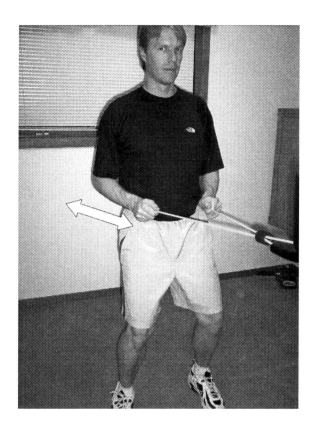

Repeat the forward/backward movements up to 50 times as tolerated.

*Remember to NEVER break the vertical plane of allowing your knee to extend beyond the toes.

6. Phase 4 is only initiated if return to sport or vocational activity require advanced rehabilitation. This phase normally continues 4 weeks beyond phase 3 rehabilitation and consists of sport specific activities and a variety of functional lifting and carrying work hardening or conditioning.

7. Sport specific functional testing may include:
    a. Stair running.
    b. Vertical jumping.
    c. Stair hopple testing
    d. Carioca/Braiding.
    e. Dot drill.
8. Some advanced or rapid rehabilitation protocols for the less invasive surgical procedures such as arthroscopy move the 4 phases of rehab from a 6 month rehab protocol to a 3 month time table with the same levels of activity as the standard rehabilitation protocols.
    a. The following rapid rehabilitation time frames are listed below:
        i.   Phase 1 occurs in 0 to 2 weeks.
        ii. Phase 2 occurs in 2 to 6 weeks.
        iii. Phase 3 occurs in 6 to 9 weeks.
        iv. Phase 4 occurs in 9 to 12 weeks.
9. Please note that some physician protocols will even shorten the above time frames into a 12 week phase 1 through 4.
    a. The key here is to remember that it takes a minimum of 6 weeks for tissue healing to occur in a healthy individual after the last trauma/micro-trauma has occurred.
    b. Post-surgically speaking, there is micro-trauma that occurs at least until full range of motion is achieved which normally occurs in the first 6 weeks of rehab.
        i. Therefore, tack on another 6 weeks and you get the justification for a 12 week rehabilitation plan.
    c. Research is all over the board with the results of 3, 4 and 6 month rehabilitation protocols regardless of the joint being operated on.
        i. Therefore, it is imperative that you use sound clinical judgment when treating and releasing your patients even when following the physician's protocol.

Chapter 10

ANKLE & FOOT

I. **General Ankle/Foot Considerations:** [3,4,32,34,47,51,58,59,63,64,70,71,80,96,104,106,113,115,123,137]

    A. The ankle and foot complex is a very complex musculo-skeletal system in the body.

        1. It consists of the Talocrural, Subtalar, Midtarsal, Tarsometatarsal, Metatarsophalangeal and Interphlanageal joints.

    B. It is important to perform a complete musculoskeletal evaluation in order to determine the correct pathology and/or symptoms before proceeding with therapeutic exercise treatment.

    C. One of the advantages with extremity evaluations is the fact that only one side is normally affected and the clinician may use the other side as a "normal" baseline.

        1. Keep in mind that a 10 percent strength differential is considered normal for the dominant hand side.

            a. For example, it would be considered normal in a right handed dominant individual to be 10 percent stronger on their dominant side.

    D. Therapeutic exercise for balanced ankle/foot rehabilitation progression:

        1. The "PRICE" principle applies for all ankle/foot rehabilitation that involves inflammation and/or trauma.

            a. "P"rotection often means refraining from sport or activity.

                a. It may also involve a neoprene or Nylon lace up brace.

            b. "R"est often means taking a break from activity.

                i. Keep in mind this excludes range of motion that requires 10 repetitions daily to maintain joint nutrition.

     Proven Therapeutic Exercise Techniques

       c.   "I"ce or cryotherapy will reduce pain and inflammation.

       d.   "C"ompression will also reduce pain and inflammation.

          Ace compression wraps and neoprene sleeves are commonly used for the ankle/foot.

       e.   "E"levation will prevent distal extremity edema and often involves laying supine or side lying on the uninvolved ankle/foot.

          i.   Sitting and standing should be minimized.

II. **Ankle/Foot Imbalances:**[3,4,32,34,47,51,58,59,63,64,70,71,80,96,104,106,109,110,113,115,123,137]

    A.   Range of motion and strength imbalances in the ankle/foot complex commonly involve the following:

       1.   Those that are typically too strong and/or tight include:

          a.   Gastrocnemius, Soleus and Plantaris causing limited dorsiflexion.

       2.   Those that are typically too weak and/or loose include:

          a.   Peroneus Longus and Brevis causing recurrent Lateral Collateral ligament ankle sprains and excessive Supination.

       3.   Those that are typically balanced include:

          a.   Tibialis Anterior, Extensor Digitorum Longus, Extensor Hallucis Longus, Tibialis Posterior, Flexor Digitorum Longus and Flexor Hallucis Longus.

       4.   It is wise to review the anatomical origins, insertions, innervations, and motions in order to fully and appropriately apply the proven therapeutic exercise techniques listed in this chapter. This information can be found in the Appendix.

III. **Ankle/Foot Reflex Mechanisms:**[3,4,32,34,47,51,58,59,63,64,70,71,80,96,104,106,113,115,123,137]

    A.   Any ankle/foot diagnosis involving pain will automatically shut down or reduce the contractility of the Peroneus Longus and Brevis muscles:

       1.   The result of this reflexive shut down causes these muscles to ineffectively resist the stresses of ankle inversion which frequently causes recurrent ankle inversion sprain/strains.

B.   Important rehabilitation considerations in the ankle/foot:
  1.   It is important to note that the Talocrural joint is triplanar.
    a.   The motion of Supination involves combination movements of plantarflexion, adduction and inversion.
    b.   The motion of Pronation involves combination movements of dorsiflexion, abduction and eversion.
  2.   Therefore, when rehabilitating recurrent lateral ankle sprain/strains it is essential to perform exercise in 3 planes of motion:
    a.   Dorsiflexion.
    b.   Abduction.
    c.   Eversion.
C.   With this information in mind, we will now take a look at specific diagnoses and proven therapeutic exercise techniques for the ankle/foot.

IV.   **Ankle/Foot Hypomobility Diagnoses and Proven Therapeutic Exercises:**[3,4,10,32,34,47,51,58,59,63,64,70,71,80,96,104, 106,113,115,123,137]

A.   Common ankle/foot hypomobility diagnoses:
  1.   Adhesive Capsulitis.
  2.   Arthritis (Osteoarthritis and Rheumatoid).
  3.   Post Surgical Rehab.
  4.   Post Fracture Rehab.
  5.   Haglan's Deformity/Achilles Bursitis.
  6.   Synovitis.
  7.   Tendonitis.
  8.   Pain.
  9.   Muscle Atrophy/Weakness.
  10.   Plantar Fasciitis.
B.   Last Minute Reminders:
  1.   Range of motion and strength deficits, or imbalances, are easily evaluated in the ankle/foot by comparing the involved side with the uninvolved ankle/foot.
C.   Proven Therapeutic Exercises for ankle/foot hypomobility:

10-1 "Ankle Stretch – Knee Straight"

Do NOT hold your breath.

Standing on a step or riser, keep your knee straight and allow the heel to drop.

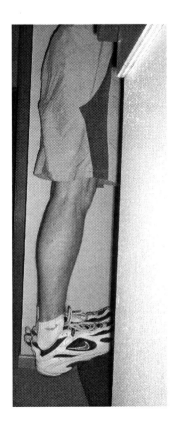

Hold the stretch position 15 to 30 seconds.

Relax and repeat 3 to 5 times as tolerated.

*This stretches the Gastrocnemius muscle primarily.

10-2 "Ankle Stretch – Knee Bent"

Do NOT hold your breath.
Standing on a step or riser, bend your knee straight 20 degrees and allow the heel to drop.

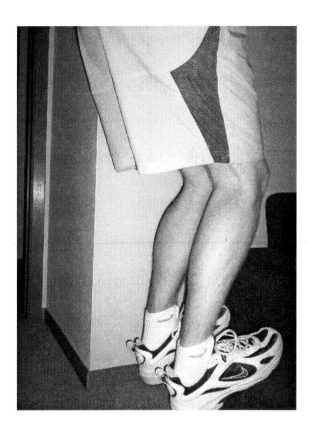

Hold the stretch position 15 to 30 seconds.
Relax and repeat 3 to 5 times as tolerated.

*This stretches the Soleus muscle primarily.

10-3 "Ankle Pumps"

Do NOT hold your breath.
Maximally dorsiflex and plantarflex your foot.

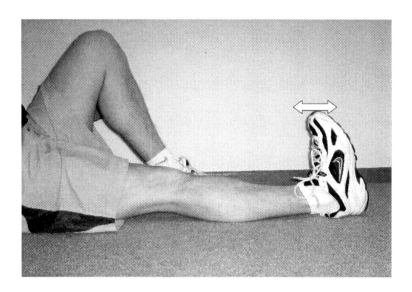

Hold 2 to 5 seconds.
Relax and repeat up to 25 times as tolerated.

10-4 "Joint Mobilizations" These are primarily performed with "anterior" mobilization force to increase plantarflexion and "posterior" mobilization force to increase dorsiflexion. Please refer to **Chapter 23** for specifics.

V. **Ankle/Foot Hypermobility Diagnoses and Proven Therapeutic Exercises:**[3,4,10,32,34,47,51,58,59,63,64,70,71,80,96,104,106,113,115,123,137]

    A.   Common ankle/foot hypermobility diagnoses:
        1.   Muscle Strains.
        2.   Ligament Sprains.
        3.   Joint Dislocations.
        4.   Anatomical Deficiencies.
        5.   Cartilage/Meniscus Tears.
        6.   Pain.
        7.   Muscle Atrophy/Weakness.
    B.   Proven Therapeutic Exercises for ankle/foot hypermobility:

10-5 "Heel Walking"

Do not hold your breath.
Walk on your heels with the toes raised up off the floor.

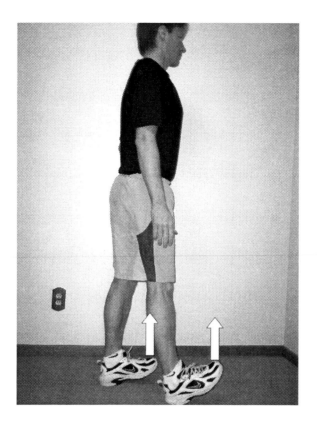

Walk at least 25 steps, break and repeat 3 to 5 times as tolerated.

10-6 "Toe Walking"

Do not hold your breath.
Walk on your toes with your heels raised up off the floor.

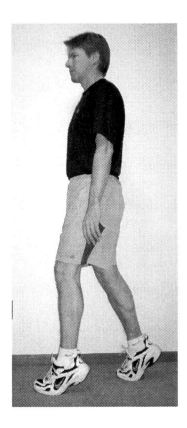

Walk at least 25 steps, break and repeat 3 to 5 times as tolerated.

10-7 "Resisted Ankle Eversion"

Do NOT hold your breath.
Evert the foot against manual resistance or a resistance band in moderate to maximal dorsiflexion.

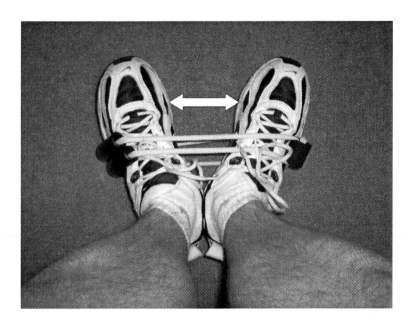

Hold 2 to 5 seconds.
Relax and repeat up to 25 times as tolerated.

10-8 "Towel Scrunches"

Do not hold your breath.
Begin with the foot flat on the floor with a towel underneath.
Keeping your heel on the floor, repetitively scrunch up the towel.

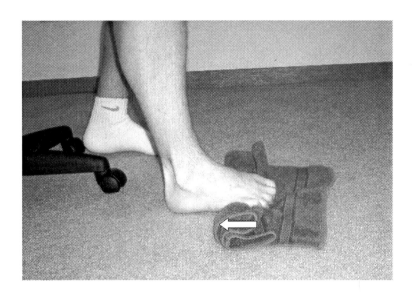

Hold 2 to 5 seconds as tolerated.
Relax and repeat up to 25 times as tolerated.

V. **Ankle/foot Neurovascular Diagnoses and Proven Therapeutic Exercises:**[3,4,10,32,34,47,51,58,59,63,64,70,71,80,96,104,106,113,115,123,137]

    A.   Common ankle/foot neurovascular diagnoses:
        1.   Reflex Sympathetic Dystrophy.
        2.   Tarsal Tunnel Syndrome.
        3.   Morton's Neuroma.
        4.   Compartment Syndrome.
        5.   Volkmann's Ischemic Contracture.
    B.   Proven Therapeutic Exercises for ankle/foot neurovascular conditions:

10-9 "Plantar Fascial Friction Stretch"

This stretch is performed by maximally dorsiflexing the ankle and toes
with one hand.

With the other hand, rub across the plantar fascia back and forth ten
times.

Progressively move up or down the plantar fascia rubbing back and
forth every finger width.

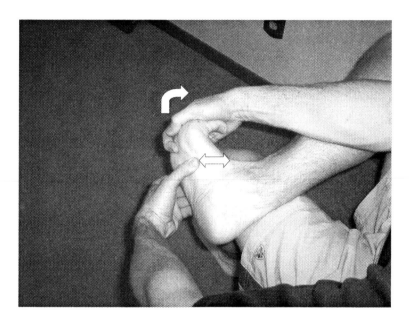

Perform back and forth movement 10 repetitions and repeat the process
3 to 5 times as tolerated.

10-10 "LLTT – Lower Limb Tissue Tension Stretch"

Do not hold your breath.
Round out the spine (if no spinal pathology contraindicates this
position).
Have the patient SLOWLY dorsiflex and plantarflex the foot 10 to
20 times as tolerated for neural flossing effects.
Pain or discomfort in the sciatic distribution along the hamstring is
normal.

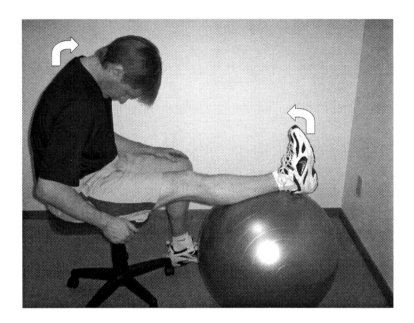

Hold 15 to 30 seconds each.
Relax and repeat 3 to 5 times as tolerated.

VII. **Ankle/foot Post Fracture/Surgical Diagnoses and Proven
    Therapeutic Exercises:** [3,4,10,13,32,34,47,51,58,59,63,64,70,71,80,96,104,106,
    113,115,123,137]

    A. Common ankle/foot post fracture/surgical diagnoses:
        1.   Ankle Arthroscopy.
        2.   Ankle/foot Muscle Repair.
        3.   Total Ankle Replacement (TAR).
        4.   Cartilage Repair.
        5.   Ligament Repair.
        6.   Ankle/Foot Fracture.

B. Proven Therapeutic Exercises for ankle/foot post fracture/surgical conditions by Brent Brotzman:
   1. It is IMPORTANT to note that these are a compilation of conservative rehabilitation measures for the afore-mentioned diagnoses.
      a. It is imperative that the treating clinician defer to the client's surgeon when treating.
   2. Collagen fibers begin to set up in 24 to 48 hours after surgery and other traumatic events.
      a. Therefore, it is imperative that the patients receive daily passive range of motion within pain tolerances of at least 10 repetitions for each involved joint and plane of motion.
   3. Phase 1 goals for weeks 0 to 6 are the gradual return to full range of motion and decreasing pain.
      a. This phase involves simple passive range of motion within pain tolerances of at least 10 repetitions for each involved joint and plane of motion.
      b. A neoprene ankle brace or heavy duty walking cast is often used after fracture/surgical intervention from 2 weeks to 6 weeks or more.
      c. Active/Resistive Exercises should be initially limited to the knee and hip as tolerated.
      d. Ankle pumps should commence as soon as tolerated to reduce the likelihood of developing a deep vein thrombosis.
      e. The hypomobility exercises listed earlier in this chapter can be initiated. See figures 10-1 through 10-4 although decreased weight bearing may be required.
      f. Pain relieving modalities are commonly used during this rehabilitation phase.
   4. Phase 2 goals for weeks 7 to 12 are full, non-painful range of motion, and increasing strength and functional activities.
      a. Active Assisted range of motion (AAROM) is initiated in the early weeks of phase 2 as pain and symptoms tolerate.
      b. Active range of motion (AROM) and light resistance isotonic (RROM) are initiated in the later weeks of phase 2 as pain and symptoms tolerate.

     c. The hypermobility exercises listed earlier in this chapter can often be initiated. See figures 10-5 through 10-8.

     d. Pain relieving modalities are used intermittently.

5. Phase 3 goals for weeks 13 to 21 are to maintain full and non-painful range of motion, improve speed and power, improve neuromuscular control, and gradually return to functional activities.

     a. Resisted Range of Motion (RROM) utilizing iso-kinetic apparatus is often performed in this phase.

          i. Eccentric activities utilizing a mini trampoline are also often performed in this phase.

     b. Functional closed chain (RROM) is also initiated in this phase as symptoms tolerate. A couple of the more efficacious exercises are listed here:

10-11 "Forward/Backward Balance Board"

Do NOT hold your breath.
Rock the balance board forward and backward in smooth fluid motion.

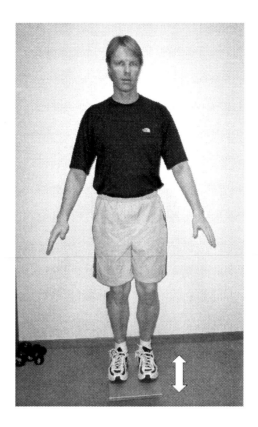

Repeat the forward/backward movements up to 50 times as tolerated.

*BAPS (Balance And Proprioreception System) boards may be used also.

10-12 "Side/Side Balance Board"

Do NOT hold your breath.
Rock the balance board side to side in smooth fluid motion.

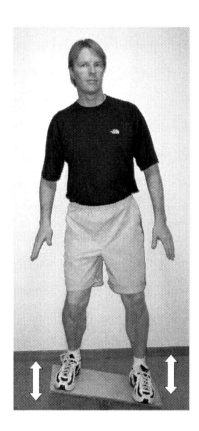

Repeat the left/right movements up to 50 times as tolerated.

*BAPS (Balance And Proprioreception System) boards may be used also.
*Circumduction movements clockwise and counterclockwise may also be used.

6.   Phase 4 is only initiated if return to sport or vocational activity require advanced rehabilitation. This phase normally continues 4 weeks beyond phase 3 rehabilitation and consists of sport specific activities and a variety of functional lifting and carrying work hardening or conditioning.

7.   Some advanced or rapid rehabilitation protocols for the less invasive surgical procedures such as arthroscopy move the 4 phases of rehab from a 6 month rehab protocol to a 4 month time table with the same levels of activity as the standard rehabilitation protocols.
     a.   The following rapid rehabilitation time frames are listed below:
          i.   Phase 1 occurs in 0 to 2 weeks.
          ii.   Phase 2 occurs in 2 to 6 weeks.
          iii. Phase 3 occurs in 6 to 12 weeks.
          iv.   Phase 4 occurs in 12 to 16 weeks.

8.   Please note that some physician protocols will even shorten the above time frames into a 12 week phase 1 through 4.
     a.   The key here is to remember that it takes a minimum of 6 weeks for tissue healing to occur in a healthy individual after the last trauma/micro-trauma has occurred.
     b.   Post-surgically speaking, there is micro-trauma that occurs at least until full range of motion is achieved which normally occurs in the first 6 weeks of rehab.
          i.   Therefore, tack on another 6 weeks and you get the justification for a 12 week rehabilitation plan.
     c.   Research is all over the board with the results of 3, 4 and 6 month rehabilitation protocols regardless of the joint being operated on.
          i.   Therefore, it is imperative that you use sound clinical judgment when treating and releasing your patients even when following the physician's protocol.

Part 4

SPINE PROVEN TECHNIQUES

Chapter 11

PROVEN THERAPEUTIC EXERCISE
TECHNIQUES–SPINE

I. **General Spinal Exercise Contraindications:**[3,4,34,44,47,51,][63,64,70,71,77,106,115,123,137]

    A. Common contraindications to active or passive exercise include, but are not limited to:
        1. Increased Inflammation.
        2. Unstable Cardio-Vascular Problems.
        3. Severe Osteoporosis.
        4. Ischemia/Peripheral Vascular Disease (PVD).
        5. Severe Pain Lasting More Than 24 Hours.
        6. Positive (+) Vertebral Artery Test for Cervical Spine Pathology.
        7. Bony Block In Spinal Range Of Motion.
        8. Infection.
        9. Fracture.
        10. Malignancy.

II. **General Spinal Exercise Precautions/Red Flags:**[3,4,34,44,][47,51,63,64,70,71,77,106,115,123,137]

    A. It is critical to follow physician protocols regarding post surgical and post fracture care with their patients.
    B. These protocols ALWAYS supercede independent treatment plans and serve to protect the treating clinician from tort or malpractice legal actions.
    C. Red Flags for possible visceral pathology (i.e., cancer) include but are not limited to:
        1. Weight Fluctuations.
        2. Inability To Sleep.
        3. Medications Are Required To Sleep.
        4. Pain Becomes Worse With Walking.
        5. Recent Fever Or Infection.

D. Other Precautions include:
    1. Delayed Onset Muscle Soreness (DOMS).
    2. Overtraining/Overwork.
    3. Severe Osteoporosis.
    4. Degree of Ischemia/Peripheral Vascular Disease (PVD).
    5. Steroid Use.
    6. Age.
    7. Avoiding Valsalva Maneuver.

III. **General Spinal Exercise Indications:**[3,4,10,34,44,47,51,63,64,70,71,77,106,112,115,123,137]

A. Common Diagnosis:
    1. Anklyosing Spondylitis (AS).
    2. Arthritis (Osteoarthritis and Rheumatoid Arthritis).
    3. Degenerative Joint Disease (DJD).
    4. Degenerative Disc Disease (DDD).
    5. Post Surgical Fusions, Laminectomies, and Microdiscectomies.
    6. Thoracic Outlet Syndrome/Thoracic Inlet Syndrome (TOS/TIS).
    7. Brachial Plexus Nerve Entrapment.
    8. Herniated Nucleus Pulposus (HNP).
    9. Facet Syndrome.
    10. Spinal Pain.
    11. Headaches.
    12. Muscle Spasms.
    13. Spinal Muscle Strains.
    14. Spinal Ligament Sprains.
    15. Brachioplexus Neuropathy.
    16. Cervical Radiculitis.
    17. Lumbar Radiculitis.
    18. Spinal Stenosis.
    19. Spondylosis.
    20. Spondylolysis.
    21. Spondylolisthesis.
    22. Retrolisthesis.
    23. Post Fracture Care.
    24. Myositis.
    25. Schmoral's Nodes.
    26. Torticollis.
    27. Scheuermann's Disease.

28. Klippel-Feil Syndrome.
29. Sprengel's Deformity.
30. Lumbago.
31. Sciatica.
32. Piriformis Syndrome.
33. Osteoporosis.
34. Sacrilization.
35. Lumbarization.
36. Spinal Tendonitis.

IV. **General Spinal Exercise Goals/Benefits:** [3,4,34,44,47,51,63, 64,70,71,77,106,115,123,137]

A. Increased Strength.
B. Increased Range of Motion.
C. Increased Flexibility.
D. Increased Endurance.
E. Increased Coordination.
F. Increased Agility.
G. Increased Balance.
H. Increased Speed.
I. Increased Stability.
J. Increased Function.
K. Decreased Pain.
L. Decreased Muscle Spasms.

V. **General Spinal Exercise Considerations:** [4,34,47,48,51,63,64,70, 71,77,83,89,99,101,103,105,109,110,112,115,128,133,139,141]

A. Spinal pain is the most common diagnosis among patients referred to physical therapy and athletic training in the United States.
   1. According to the statistics, 80 percent of adults will have at least one episode of spinal pain that requires professional evaluation and treatment in their lifetime. [19,25]
   2. Unless you are in a specialty clinic that does not treat any spinal pain, you will see a majority of patients with some form of spinal pain diagnosis.
B. The principles of efficacious spinal rehabilitation exercises are well-founded and researched, yet the application of spinal stabilization into a treatment plan is often overlooked.
   1. All too often, treatment providers of spinal pain provide modalities, massage, stretching, and a few strengthening exercises for good measure.

2. These treatments generally work as 90 percent of spinal pain episodes subside within six weeks of conservative treatment including the aforementioned treatments.
3. But, how many of these patients will have repetitive episodes of spinal pain/injury over the course of a year? Over the course of their lifetime? What about the 10 percent of spinal pain episodes that do not subside within six weeks of conservative care?
4. We have all seen, and possibly dreaded, the chronic spinal pain patient who often floats from clinic to clinic in search of a panacea for their pain.
5. What can we offer these patients as a potentially long-term solution to their pain? For that matter, what can we offer the 90 percent of patients that have episodic spinal pain?
6. The answer is NEUTRAL SPINAL STABILIZATION!

VI. **Neutral Spine Concept:** [4,34,47,48,51,63,64,70,71,77,83,89,99,101,103,105, 109,110,112,115,128,133,139,141]

A. The concept of a "NEUTRAL SPINE" is the key to successful spinal rehabilitation.
1. Any spinal diagnosis will respond favorably to neutral spinal stabilization exercises because of the neutral stresses they place on the spine.
   a. Whereas, certain diagnoses respond best from McKenzie Extension exercises like Herniated Nucleus Pulposus' (HNP's), Sprain/Strains, Retrolisthesis in the Lumbar spine.
   b. Yet other diagnoses respond best from the application of Williams Flexion exercises like Stenosis, Spondylolysis, Spondylolisthesis in the Lumbar spine.
      i. These will be covered later in the section.
B. We want to emphasize that Neutral Spinal Stabilization is a tool to be used by clinicians in the treatment of spinal pain.
1. We are not advocating the abandonment of modalities, massage, manual therapy techniques, acupuncture, or any other form of researched treatment.
2. This is simply another tool in our toolbox that will help us heal patients with spinal pain.
C. Many of the concepts and techniques that we will talk about have come from the following works:

1. Muscle Imbalances: Kendall and Sahrman.
2. Reflex Mechanisms: Richardson and Hodges.
3. Neural Tissue Extensibility: Saunders.

VII. **Muscle Imbalances in the Spine:**[62,109,110]
   A. This section is largely based on the research works by Florence Kendall and Shirley Sahrman and these renowned therapists introduced me to the concept of muscle imbalances back in 1993.
      1. What I learned from their research is the fact that muscle imbalances can occur from front to back (anteriorly to posteriorly) or right to left.
   B. Muscle imbalances can result from a myriad of different reasons:
      1. Dominant versus non-dominant sides.
      2. Pain and/or muscle spasms.
      3. Incorrect strengthening and stretching exercises.
         a. We are all familiar with the weight lifter at the gym who continuously works on the glamour muscles; biceps, pectorals, and quadriceps, but who ignores the back muscles, hamstrings, and calf muscles.
         b. The result is a typical anterior muscle imbalance which rounds out the upper back into extreme kyphosis and often causes some type of spinal pain.
   C. Most muscle imbalances are easily seen upon initial evaluation.
      1. Strength or flexibility differences between right and left or front to back are usually easy to pick up.
      2. These imbalances create torsional or shear forces which are constant on the spine, resulting in pain, and muscle spasms most frequently.
      3. Muscle imbalances also compromise the healing of an injured spinal tissue because of the constant imbalance stresses.
   D. The Body In Balance:
      1. The following represents the anterior to posterior strength ratios that are considered normal in the human body and minimize spinal stresses and anytime these strength ratios are imbalanced, pain and compromised healing is likely to result.
      2. Most of these strength ratios are well researched and based on standard normal population groups: [11,16,24,28]

      a. Cervical Flexors are $^2/_3$ as strong as Cervical Extensors.

      b. Thoracic Extensors are $^2/_3$ as strong as Thoracic Flexors.

      c. Lumbar Flexors are $^2/_3$ as strong as Lumbar Extensors.

      d. Hamstrings are $^2/_3$ as strong as Quadriceps.

VIII. **Neutral Spinal Stabilization:** [105]

  A. Neutral Spinal Stabilization is a proven system of therapeutic exercise that is well founded in research, and something that I have personally applied to thousands of patients suffering from spinal pain since 1993.

  B. It works! In fact, I have found that it works for every patient with ANY type of spinal pain resulting from ANY diagnosis in which therapeutic exercise is not contraindicated.

  C. If this sounds like a guarantee, it is as long as the principles and techniques of this course are followed, and combined with sound clinical and professional judgment, it will work.

  D. Of course, every professional must also follow contraindications to therapeutic exercise to ensure patient safety.

      1. While a patient's pain may not completely resolve, it empowers patients with knowledge and techniques they can utilize throughout their life.

Chapter 12

PROVEN CERVICAL SPINE EXERCISES

I. **Cervical Spine Imbalances:**[4,34,47,48,51,63,64,70,71,77,83,89,99,101,103,105,109,110,112,115,119,128,133,139,141]

A. How To Test Strength Imbalances in the Cervical Spine:
1. The cervical flexors should be about $\frac{2}{3}$ as strong as the cervical extensors.
    a. This may be tested manually with a force dynamometer in the healthy patient population.
    b. However, patients with neck pain generally do not like the pressure of the dynamometer placed on their head.
2. A better and more consistent way to test the balance employs a strength and endurance combination test.
    a. If you have access to an isotonic neck extension machine and neck flexion machine, you may test the patient by having them perform repetitive neck extension at approximately 10 percent of the patient's body weight until fatigued. Then test neck flexion at $\frac{2}{3}$ of the neck extension weight until fatigued.
        i. For example, a 200 pound patient performed 35 repetitions of neck extension at 20 pounds with fatigue. Then the patient performed 35 repetitions of neck flexion at 14 pounds with fatigue. This example is a patient who has a normal cervical muscle balance anteriorly/posteriorly.
    b. The problem with this method is the fact that if a patient has neck pain, spasms or a diagnosis that becomes worse with repetitive flexion or extension this test is skewed and invalid.

179

    i. Therefore, this test is best for the healthy back population.
  3. Many patients will not tolerate either of the aforementioned tests if they have significant neck back pain, and it is difficult to test. However, one way that may be tolerated includes prone spinal extension in which the forehead is held at a level of one inch above the mat table for a measured period of time. Then the cervical flexor strength/endurance is tested supine with the back of the head held one inch above the mat table for a measured period of time.
    a. For example, if the patient holds cervical extension for one minute; he or she should be able to hold cervical flexion for about 40 seconds to be in balance.
 B. Common Muscle Imbalances of the Cervical Spine:
  1. More often than not, the neck extensors (i.e., Erector Spinae group) are much stronger than the neck flexors (i.e., Sternocleidomastoid, Longus Colli) than the 1 : ⅔ ratio.
 C. How To Test Muscle Flexibility Imbalances of The Cervical Spine:
  1. Right to left imbalances of spinal flexibility are easily found with goniometric or inclinometric range of motion measurements.
    a. However, many flexibility limitations measured may be due to segmental blocks or facet blocks, or pain.
 D. Common Flexibility Imbalances of the Cervical Spine:
  1. Most often I have found that the Upper Trapezius and Scalene muscles are imbalanced and tight.
    a. When these muscles are tight bilaterally, they create a compression force on the cervical spine which reduces disc height and nerve root clearance.
    b. When these muscles are imbalanced and tight unilaterally they create a unilateral compression force on the cervical spine compromising the nerve and nerve root clearance on the side which is found to be tight.

       c.   When the Scalenes are tight, brachial plexus compression can also result which may increase distal radiating signs and symptoms.

       d.   Those patients with excessive forward head positioning almost always have tight Upper Traps and Scalenes.

2.   The best way I have found to test the flexibility of the Scalenes is to passively side bend the head while depressing the shoulder blade. Most often patients are able to best relax in the supine position. The distance from the ear to the Acromioclavicular joint should be recorded.

       a.   The test is performed left and right. The distance from the shoulder left to right should not exceed 10 percent, or an imbalance is indicated.

       b.   Often the patient will also tell you which side felt tighter.

3.   The best way I have found to test the flexibility of the Upper Trapezius is to passively side bend and flex/rotate the head forward. Most often patients are able to best relax in the supine position or the sitting position. The distance from the chin to the Acromioclavicular joint should be recorded.

       a.   The test is performed left and right and the distance from the Acromioclavicular joint left to right should not exceed 10 percent or a muscle imbalance is indicated.

II. **Cervical Spine Reflex Mechanisms:** [105]

    A.   Largely based on the research works of Richardson and Hodges. This spinal research group in Queensland, Australia has been sticking patients with electromyography (EMG) needles who suffer from neck pain for several years.

       1.   The results of their studies have found that any legitimate cervical spine pain will automatically shut down the Longus Colli muscles of the cervical spine.

       2.   Remember, the Longus Colli muscles are spinal stabilizers and occupy the space on the anterior surface of the cervical vertebrae.

           a.   They contribute very little to cervical flexion, less than 5 percent.

   b. However, they contribute a significant amount to stabilizing the cervical spine (i.e., over 40 percent).

B. What happens when the Longus Colli muscles shut down?

  1. The Semispinalis, Splenius, and Upper Trapezius now have 2 jobs:

   a. They are responsible for moving the cervical spine, primarily for extension.

   b. And, now they must also try and stabilize the cervical spine.

    i. This over stresses the Semispinalis, Splenius, and Upper Trapezius and causing pain, spasms, and fatigue.

C. The Australian research group, Richardson and Hodges, has shown that in order to rehabilitate the Longus Colli muscles we must employ the Chin Tuck exercise.

  1. Chin tucks automatically or reflexively contract the Longus Colli muscles allowing them to strengthen.

   a. The Chin Tuck is the key and cornerstone to cervical stabilization. (See Figure 12-1)

   b. Chin tucks should be performed prior to any other cervical strengthening exercises.

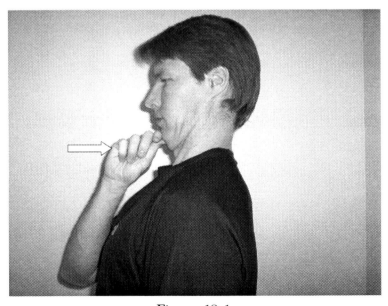

Figure 12-1

2. The multi-faceted benefits of chin tucks:
    a. Chin tucks also increase the amount of space between the occiput and C2 spinous process.
       i. This space is often referred to as the suboccipital space.
       ii. This space should be about one finger width wide.
       iii. If the space is less that one finger width wide, the Greater and Lesser Occipital Nerves that pass through this area can become impinged or entrapped, causing occipital headaches.
       iv. Occipital headaches are often referred to as stress or tension headaches, because stress increases the suboccipital muscle tone decreasing the amount of space for the occipital nerves.
3. When performing chin tucks, make sure that the Sternocleidomastoid muscle does not contract.
    a. This muscle is easy to palpate during chin tuck exercises to ensure its flaccidity.

D. Another frequent cause of headaches among patients with cervical spine traumatic injuries is Temporal Mandibular Joint dysfunction.
1. The Temporal Mandibular Joint (TMJ) is the only bilateral joint in the body.
    a. If one side of the TMJ is injured, it will affect the kinematics of both sides.
    b. This often causes bilateral jaw pain which can manifest itself as headaches.
    c. A quick evaluation of the TMJ joints is required before accurately treating a patient with neck pain.

E. The Vertebral Artery Test MUST be performed before significant evaluation and/or treatment of the cervical spine can be performed.
1. The Vertebral Artery Test is performed as follows:
    a. The patient keeps their eyes open and gazing forward while the clinician gently and slowly extends and rotates the neck/head to one side, holding 10 seconds. Repeat on both sides.
2. If the vertebral artery test causes dizziness or nystagmus of the eye(s), it contraindicates most forms of treatment

and needs to be referred back to the physician for appropriate care.

III. **Cervical Spine Nerve Extensibility:** [112]
   A. Duane Saunders is a pioneer in developing eclectic spinal evaluations and treatment approaches. According to his research and works, nerve extensibility is the most often overlooked evaluative technique in the cervical spine.
   B. The brachial plexus can become impinged between the following structures:
      1. Scalenes (muscle spasms or tightness).
      2. The Clavicle.
      3. The Pectoralis Minor muscle.
         a. Any of these structures that impinge the brachial plexus can cause distal radicular signs and symptoms.
         b. Patients generally refer to their whole hand tingling or numb.
            i. This may also be referred to as Thoracic Outlet or Inlet Syndrome (TOS or TIS).
   C. However, the brachial plexus may also be entrapped at the exit of the nerve root from the vertebral foramen.
      1. As many spinal injuries heal, the healing process lays down collagen and elastin fibers to scar or reinforce the injured area.
      2. Unfortunately some of this scarring lays down spider web like fibers attaching the spinal nerve root to the dural sleeve or to the spinal vertebral foramen.
         a. This reduces the mobility of the nerve, dura, and often entraps or limits the nerve root migration with spinal movements thus causing pain.
   D. How to Test for Upper Limb Tissue Tension/Brachial Plexus Extensibility:
      1. This test must be performed very carefully, and it is NOT recommended for patients with HNP diagnoses.
      2. Lay the patient supine and side bend and rotate the head to one direction. Provide simultaneous shoulder blade distraction to the side opposite of the head rotation. Have the patient slowly extend the arm with the palm up. Then have the patient slowly extend the wrist and fingers to maximum tolerance. If pain and repro-

duction of symptoms occur upon the test, the brachial plexus extensibility is limited. If the patient is unable to fully extend the wrist and fingers, brachial plexus extensibility is limited. This test specifically isolates the median nerve with nerve roots C5-8. Test left, and right arms separately. (See Figure 12-2)

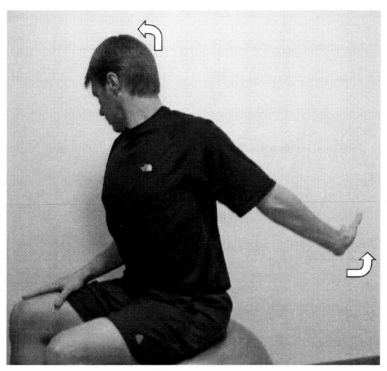

Figure 12-2

E. How To Improve Brachial Plexus Extensibility:
    1. Brachial plexus extensibility is improved the same way you tested for it. Have the patient hold each stretch 15 to 20 seconds and repeat 3 to 5 times. As the symptoms improve, you may have them alternately flex and extend the wrist and fingers often referred to as "Neural Flossing." This is very difficult to have patients perform independently, and generally requires the assistance of a trained clinician.

IV. **Neutral Cervical Spine Stabilization Exercises:** [4,34,47,48,]
[51,63,64,70,71,77,83,89,99,101,103,105,109,110,112,115,128,133,139,141]

A. Cervical stabilization employs the concept of a neutral spine.
   1. Make sure the neutral cervical spine positioning is maintained for all exercises.
   2. Cervical stabilization follows a defined sequence from easy to hard.
   3. Most patients begin with 5 to 10 exercises, and progress 5 repetitions per week to a maximum of 25 repetitions for each exercise.
   4. We do not recommend any continuous repetitions over 25 repetitions because of the risk of overuse injury or tendonitis.
B. Stretches for muscle imbalances or nerve imbalances should be performed BEFORE cervical stabilization to minimize inadvertent spinal stresses.
   1. Exercises for muscle weakness imbalances should also be performed BEFORE cervical stabilization to minimize inadvertent spinal stresses.
C. Modalities such as superficial heat, cold, ultrasound, electrical stimulation and cervical traction may be performed before or after cervical stabilization exercises depending on the clinician's purpose, and of course as long as they are NOT contraindicated.
D. Level 1 Cervical Stabilization is the cornerstone of all advanced levels of stabilization.
   1. The Chin Tuck exercise should be performed before initiating any level 2 to 5 exercise and held throughout the exercise.
   2. Most cervical stabilization exercises should be held 2 to 5 seconds, and repeated up to 25 repetitions as long as the neutral spine is not compromised.
   3. The Chin Tuck is performed by the following command:
      a. "Push your chin straight back, do not lift or flex your head forward, keep your eyes focused on something straight ahead of you . Do not hold your breath." (See Figure 12-1)
   4. Positions To Perform Chin Tucks:
      a. ALL positions: supine, prone, four point, tall kneeling, standing, and sitting are appropriate.

b.   Supine is the preferred position to initially instruct patients on the exercise because it is easiest to relax the Sternocleidomastoid (SCM) muscles.

3.   How long do you hold the Chin Tuck contraction?

a.   At least 10 seconds, for 20 to 30 repetitions.

i.   Ten seconds of contraction generally allows patients enough time to complete brief lifting tasks in which the Longus Colli will maximize stability to the cervical spine and reducing the possibility of injury.

4.   How do you know when the Longus Colli is of normal strength?

a.   Based on empirical data that I have collected on thousands of patients with neck pain, I have found the best way to establish a baseline and follow-up measurement is to have the patient lie supine with a folded up blood pressure cuff under the nape of the cervical spine. Pump up the cuff up to 20 mmHG. Instruct the patient to elongate the neck and push the cervical spine flat. Do not allow the patient to hold their breath. Record the blood pressure cuff measurement upon initial instruction, then upon discharge or re-evaluation to chart progress.

i.   I have found that most baseline measures in patients with neck pain ranges from 2 to 4 mmHG increase in pressure.

ii. I have found that in patients with no neck pain, or in those who have resolved their neck pain that the pressure in the cuff increases to 10 or more mmHG upon chin tuck contraction.

iii. Unfortunately, this does tend to fluctuate in patients with limited cervical mobility, and does not represent a standard, but rather a generality.

iv. This is empirical data that I have measured and recorded over the since 1995 and should be useful to you in writing functional outcome oriented goals, (i.e., "Increase Longus Colli Strength of contraction to 10 mmHG by 6 weeks in order to decrease pain and spasms to resume normal work duties of lifting up to 20 pounds on a 'frequent' basis without exacerbation of symptoms.")

    5. Longus Colli muscle strengthening is the cornerstone of cervical stabilization and functional lifting.

        a. Therefore, the Chin Tuck exercise needs to be voluntarily performed before any of the cervical stabilization exercises or before any functional lifting activities such as work conditioning or work hardening.

        b. Remember, as long as there is any neck pain, the Longus Colli will not stabilize the cervical spine due to reflex shut down.

E. QUALITY of the neutral cervical stabilization exercises are paramount to the QUANTITY of exercises.

F. As you progress a patient through the levels of stabilization, it is NOT necessary to continue the previous level's exercises as they are largely incorporated into the next level of exercise.

    1. However, there may be times where multiple levels of spinal stabilization exercises need to be performed.

G. The following Cervical Stabilization Exercises are not all inclusive, however they represent exercises that will NOT create muscular imbalances in strength or flexibility.

    1. These exercises also work all major muscle groups contributing to the stability of the cervical spine.

    2. Some of these exercises will be presented in the Thoracic and or Lumbar Spinal Stabilization sections as they contribute to spinal stability in those areas as well.

H. There is an old saying in rehabilitation that goes: "Proximal Stability for Distal Mobility."

    1. Many of the cervical stabilization exercises involve working the scapular muscles.

    2. The stronger the scapular muscles, the less stress that will occur in the cervical spine.

    3. In fact, many of these scapular muscles originate in the thoracic spine and attach to the cervical spine or skull. Therefore, some overlap will exist in these stability exercises for the cervical and thoracic spines.

4. Recommended advanced exercises:
    a. There are two excellent resources for advanced
        spinal stabilization utilizing the Foam Roller and
        Swiss Ball apparatus by author Caroline Creager,
        PT and can be purchased at: OPTP Publications,
        1-800-367-7393 or web site *www.optp.com.*

LEVEL 1 CERVICAL STABILIZATION:

12-1 "Chin Tuck"

Do not hold your breath.
Push your chin straight back/elongate the neck
Keep your eyes focused straight ahead.

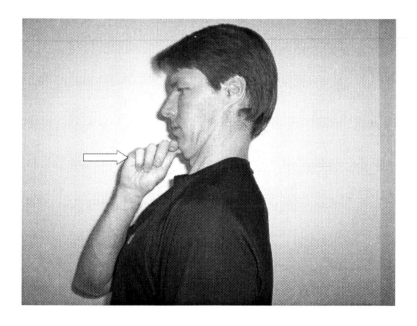

Hold >10 seconds as tolerated.
Relax and repeat 20 to 30 times as tolerated.

12-3 "Chin Tuck with Cervical Flexion"

Do not hold your breath.
Perform the chin tuck and hold the position.
Lift the head 1 to 2 inches off the floor/plinth in 2 to 5 seconds.

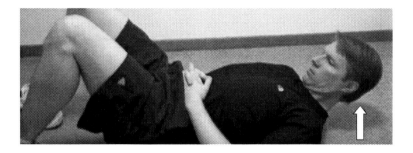

Relax and repeat up to 25 times as tolerated.

*Do not progress to level 2 unless symptoms are minimal.

LEVEL 2 CERVICAL STABILIZATION

12-4 "4 Way Cervical Isometrics"

Do not hold your breath.
Perform the chin tuck and hold the position.
Firmly press against both hands in all 4 quadrant positions.

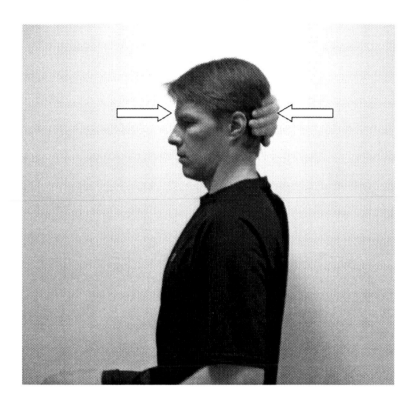

Hold 2 to 5 seconds.
Relax and repeat up to 25 times as tolerated.
Make sure you do NOT move your head.

*You may use oblique angles of isometric resistance if pure planar motion resistance is not tolerated.
*Do not progress to Level 3 unless symptoms are minimal.

LEVEL 3 CERVICAL STABILIZATION

12-5 "Resisted Scapular External Rotation"

Do not hold your breath.
Perform the chin tuck and hold the position.
Keep your elbows at your side at all times.
Pull the resistance band apart and hold 2 to 5 seconds.

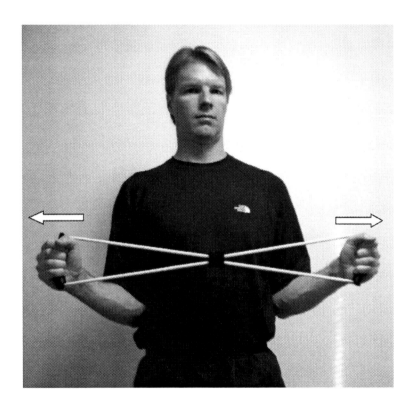

Relax and repeat up to 25 times as tolerated.

12-6 "Resisted Scapular Extension"

Do not hold your breath.
Perform the chin tuck and hold the position.
Keel your elbows straight
Pull the resistance band back and hold 2 to 5 seconds.

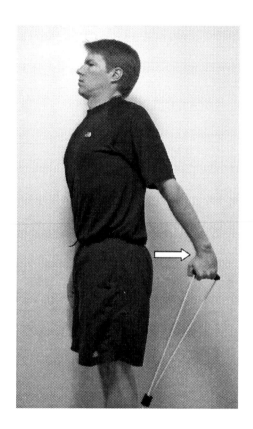

Relax and repeat up to 25 times as tolerated.

*Do not progress to Level 4 unless symptoms are minimal.

LEVEL 4 CERVICAL STABILIZATION

12-7 "4 Point Arm Extension"

Do not hold your breath.
Perform the chin tuck and hold the position.
Keep your elbows straight.
Lift your arm straight in front of you and hold 2 to 5 seconds.

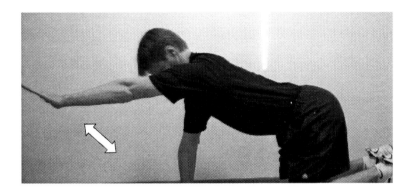

Relax and repeat up to 25 times as tolerated.

12-8 "Saws"

Do not hold your breath.
Perform the chin tuck and hold the position.

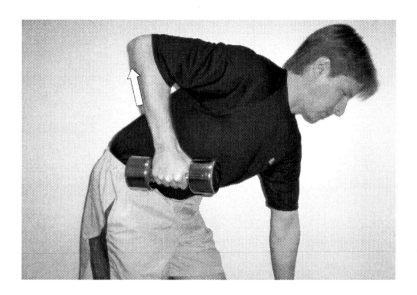

Pull the arm back and hold 2 to 5 seconds.
Relax and repeat up to 25 times as tolerated.

*May use resistance bands or dumbbell weights to increase resistance.
*Do not progress to Level 5 unless symptoms are minimal.

LEVEL 5 CERVICAL STABILIZATION

12-9 "4 Point 1 Arm Saws"

Do not hold your breath.
Perform the chin tuck and hold the position.
Stabilize your forehead on the Swiss ball.
Pull the arm back and hold 2 to 5 seconds.

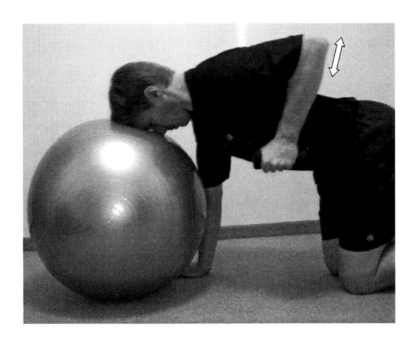

Relax and repeat up to 25 times as tolerated.

*May use resistance bands or dumbbell weights to increase resistance.

12-10 "4 Point 2 Arm Saws"

Do not hold your breath.
Perform the chin tuck and hold the position.
Stabilize your forehead on the Swiss ball.
Pull both arms back and hold 2 to 5 seconds.

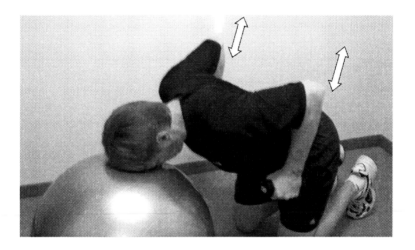

Relax and repeat up to 25 times as tolerated.

*May use resistance bands or dumbbell weights to increase resistance.

Chapter 13

PROVEN THORACIC SPINE EXERCISES

I. **Thoracic Spine Imbalances:** [4,34,47,48,51,63,64,70,71,77,83,89,99,101,
    103,105,109,110,112,115,119,133,139,141]

A. How To Test Strength Imbalances in the Thoracic Spine:
    1. The thoracic extensors should be about $\frac{2}{3}$ as strong as
        the thoracic flexors.
        a. This is difficult to test manually with a force
            dynamometer.
    2. A common flaw of testing these muscles is to test bench
        press for thoracic flexor strength.
        a. The problem with this test is the fact that the tri-
            ceps contribute significant force for the bench press
            activity, but do not contribute the thoracic flexor
            strength.
    3. A better and more consistent way to test the balance
        employs a strength and endurance combination test us-
        ing the isotonic rowing machine to test thoracic exten-
        sion, and a pectoral fly machine (Pec Deck) to test tho-
        racic flexion.
        a. If you have access to these machines, have the pa-
            tient perform repetitive pectoral flexion/adduction
            at approximately 25 percent of the patient's body
            weight until fatigued. Then test thoracic extension
            with the rowing machine at $\frac{2}{3}$ of the thoracic flex-
            ion weight until fatigued.
            i. For example, a 200 pound patient performed
                35 repetitions of thoracic flexion (Pec Deck)
                at 50 pounds with fatigue. Then the patient
                performed 35 repetitions of neck flexion at
                30 pounds with fatigue. This example is a pa-
                tient who has a normal muscle balance anteri-
                orly/posteriorly.

   b. The problem with this method is the fact that if a patient has upper back pain, spasms or a diagnosis that becomes worse with repetitive flexion or extension this test is skewed and invalid.

     i. Therefore, this test is best for the healthy back population.

  4. Unfortunately, many patients will not tolerate either of the aforementioned tests if they have significant upper back pain, and it is difficult to test.

   a. There is NOT a sufficiently valid or reliable test of a muscle imbalance for these types of patients in the research literature.

   b. However, we may manually muscle test the patient's thoracic flexors or extensors and give a less quantitative grade to the degree of imbalance.

B. Common Muscle Imbalances of the Thoracic Spine:

  1. Most often the thoracic flexors (Pectorals, Anterior Deltoid, Biceps) are much stronger than the thoracic extensors (Rhomboids, Middle Trapezius) than the $1 : \frac{2}{3}$ ratio.

C. How To Test Muscle Flexibility Imbalances of the Thoracic Spine:

  1. Right to left imbalances of spinal flexibility are easily found with goniometric or inclinometric range of motion measurements.

   a. However, many flexibility limitations measured may be due to segmental blocks or facet blocks, or pain.

   b. There is also much less segmental motion of the thoracic spine due to the rib articulations.

D. Common Flexibility Imbalances of the Thoracic Spine:

  1. Most often I have found that the Pectoralis Major and Minor muscles are imbalanced and tight.

   a. When these muscles are tight bilaterally, they create an anterior traction force on the thoracic spine.

   b. When these muscles are imbalanced and tight unilaterally, they create a unilateral anterior torsional force on the thoracic spine and surrounding musculature often compromising nerve and nerve root clearance on the side which is found to be tight.

      i.   Unilateral muscle imbalances often occur on the dominant hand side of the patient.

    c. Either condition may also result in pain, muscle spasms, or radicular signs in the upper extremities.

2. The best way I have found to test the flexibility of the Pectoralis Major and Minor muscles is to perform the High Corner Stretch. (Figure 13-1)

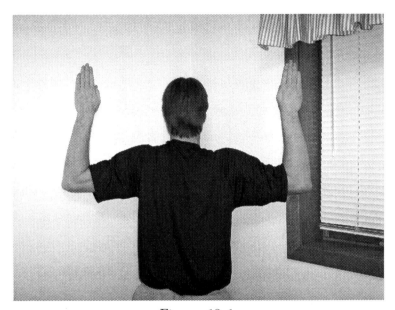

Figure 13-1

    a. This stretch is performed by the patient placing one arm on each wall in a corner with the forearm (elbow to wrist) laying completely flat on the wall.

       i.   You will be able to see tightness left to right or bilaterally based on the anterior/posterior position of the Humerus in relation to the elbow.

       ii. If the head of the Humerus is unable to assume a position anterior to the elbow, it is considered tight.

       iii. The anterior/posterior distance from one Humeral head to the elbow should NOT exceed 10 percent from right to left or an imbalance is indicated. Often the patient will also tell you which side felt tighter.

II. **Thoracic Spine Reflex Mechanisms:** [105]
   A. Largely based on the research works of Richardson and Hodges. This spinal research group in Queensland, Australia has been sticking patients with electromyography (EMG) needles who suffer from spinal pain for several years.
      1. The results of their studies have found that any legitimate thoracic spine pain will automatically shut down the Rhomboids muscles of the thoracic spine.
      2. Remember, the Rhomboids muscles are spinal stabilizers and occupy the space between the medial surfaces of the scapula to the spinous processes of T1-6.
         a. They contribute very little to thoracic extension, less than 5 percent.
         b. However, they contribute a significant amount to stabilizing the thoracic spine, (i.e., over 45 percent).
   B. What happens when the Rhomboid muscles shut down?
      1. The Erector Spinae group now has 2 jobs:
         a. They are responsible for moving the thoracic spine, primarily for extension.
         b. And now they must also try and stabilize the thoracic spine.
            i. This over stresses the Erector Spinae group in addition to the Upper Trapezius and Levator Scapulae muscles causing pain, spasms, and fatigue.
   C. The Australian research group has shown that in order to effectively and efficiently rehabilitate the Rhomboid muscles we must employ the Shoulder Squeeze exercise.
      1. Shoulder Squeezes automatically or reflexively contract the Rhomboid Major and Minor muscles allowing them to strengthen.
      2. The Shoulder Squeeze is the key and cornerstone to thoracic stabilization.
         a. Shoulder squeezes should be performed prior to any other cervical strengthening exercises. (See Figure 13-2)

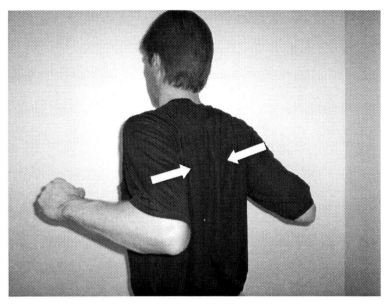

Figure 13-2

    b.   In order to perform this exercise correctly the patient must NOT over contract the Rhomboids.
        i.   If this occurs you will see shoulder elevation because the Upper Trapezius and Levator Scapulae muscles will over-power the Rhomboids.
        ii.   It is more of a 'setting' exercise to be performed prior to any level of thoracic stabilization.

III. **Thoracic Spine Nerve Extensibility:**[113]
    A.   Duane Saunders is a pioneer in developing eclectic spinal evaluations and treatment approaches. According to his research and works, nerve extensibility is the most often overlooked evaluative technique in the thoracic spine.
    B.   The brachial plexus can become impinged between the following structures:
        1.   Scalenes (muscle spasms or tightness).
        2.   The Clavicle.
        3.   The Pectoralis Minor muscle.
            a.   Any of these structures that impinge the brachial plexus can cause distal radicular signs and symptoms.

        i.   Patients generally refer to their whole hand tingling or numb.

        ii.   This may also be referred to as Thoracic Outlet or Inlet Syndrome (TOS or TIS).

    4.   Although we also test this in the cervical spine and shoulder pathologies, it also needs to be tested in the thoracic spine evaluation because of the overlapping structures that can involve the brachial plexus.

C.   The brachial plexus may also be entrapped at the exit of the nerve root from the vertebral foramen.

    1.   As many spinal injuries heal, the healing process lays down collagen and elastin fibers to scar or reinforce the injured area.

    2.   Unfortunately some of this scarring lays down spider web like fibers attaching the spinal nerve root to the dural sleeve or to the spinal vertebral foramen.

        a.   This reduces the mobility of the nerve, dura, and often entraps or limits the nerve root migration with spinal movements thus causing pain.

D.   How to Test for Upper Limb Tissue Tension/Brachial Plexus Extensibility:

    1.   This test must be performed very carefully, and it is NOT recommended for patients with HNP diagnoses.

    2.   Lay the patient supine and side bend and rotate the head to one direction. Provide simultaneous shoulder blade distraction to the side opposite of the head rotation. Have the patient slowly extend the arm with the palm up. Then have the patient slowly extend the wrist and fingers to maximum tolerance. If pain and reproduction of symptoms occur upon the test, the brachial plexus extensibility is limited. If the patient is unable to fully extend the wrist and fingers, brachial plexus extensibility is limited. This test specifically isolates the median nerve with nerve roots C5-8. Test left, and right arms separately. (See Figure 12-2)

E.   How To Improve Brachial Plexus Extensibility:

    1.   Brachial plexus extensibility is improved the same way you tested for it. Have the patient hold each stretch 15 to 20 seconds and repeat 3 to 5 times. As the symptoms improve, you may have them alternately flex and ex-

tend the wrist and fingers often referred to as "Neural Flossing." This is very difficult to have patients perform independently, and generally requires the assistance of a trained clinician.

IV. **Commonly Overlooked Thoracic Spine Conditions:**[4,34, 47,48,51,63,64,70,71,77,83,89,99,101,103,105,109,110,112,115,128,133,139,141]

   A.   The Clay Shoveler's Fracture is an occult fracture of the Transverse or Spinous Process of a thoracic vertebrae.

      1.   This fracture is very difficult to see on plain film x-rays and often presents as chronic sharp and stabbing upper back pain.

      2.   If symptoms do NOT improve in 6 to 8 weeks of conservative care, you should consider this a possibility depending on the mechanism of injury.

   B.   Ankylosing Spondylitis (AS) is a stiff spine caused by degeneration of the vertebrae.

      1.   The test parameters for this diagnosis are to measure the rib cage circumferentially at the nipple line for males and below the bust line for females while standing.

      2.   Measurements are taken and recorded with full inhalation and exhalation.

      3.   If the difference in measurements is less than 2 inches, AS is suspect.

V. **Neutral Thoracic Spine Stabilization Exercises:**[4,34,47,48, 51,63,64,70,71,77,83,89,99,101,103,105,109,110,112,115,128,133,139,141]

   A.   Thoracic stabilization employs the concept of a neutral spine.

      1.   Make sure the neutral thoracic spine is maintained for all exercises.

      2.   Thoracic stabilization follows a defined sequence from easy to hard.

      3.   Most patients begin with 5 to 10 exercises, and progress 5 repetitions per week to a maximum of 25 repetitions for each exercise.

      4.   We do not recommend any continuous repetitions over 25 repetitions because of the risk of overuse injury or tendonitis.

   B.   Stretches for muscle imbalances or nerve imbalances should be performed before thoracic stabilization to minimize inadvertent spinal stresses.

      1.   Exercises for muscle weakness imbalances should also be performed before thoracic stabilization to minimize inadvertent spinal stresses.

C.   Modalities such as superficial heat, cold, ultrasound, electrical stimulation and diathermy may be performed before or after thoracic stabilization exercises depending on the clinician s purpose, and of course as long as they are NOT contraindicated.

D.   Level 1 Thoracic Stabilization is the cornerstone of all advanced levels of stabilization.

      1.   The Shoulder Squeeze should be performed before initiating any level 2 to 5 exercise and held throughout the exercise.

      2.   Most thoracic stabilization exercises should be held 2 to 5 seconds, and repeated up to 25 repetitions as long as the neutral spine position is not compromised.

      3.   The Shoulder Squeeze is performed by the following command, "Pull your shoulders back and pinch the shoulder blades together. Do not hold your breath." (See Figure 13-2)

      4.   Positions To Perform Shoulder Squeezes:

           a.   ALL positions: supine, prone, four point, tall kneeling, standing, and sitting are appropriate.

           b.   Sitting or standing is the preferred position to initially instruct patients on the exercise because it is easiest to relax the Upper Trapezius muscles.

               i.   If the Upper Trapezius and Levator Scapulae muscles are contracted, shoulder elevation will result which does NOT contribute to neutral thoracic stabilization techniques or goals.

      3.   How long do you hold the Shoulder Squeeze contraction?

           a.   At least 10 seconds, for 20 to 30 repetitions.

               i.   Ten seconds of contraction generally allows patients enough time to complete brief lifting tasks in which the Rhomboid Major and Minor will maximize stability to the thoracic spine and reduce the possibility of injury.

      4.   How do you know when the Rhomboids are of normal strength?

    a.   This is difficult to test, however one way to test is a combination strength and endurance test in which the patient will perform repetitive Scapular Retraction, usually with a rowing machine or similar apparatus, until fatigue.

    b.   Empirically, I have tested and kept records on over 2,000 patients. The results include a 50 repetition fatigue at 20 percent of the patient's body weight in normal, healthy adults without mid-back pain.

        i.   For example, if a 200 pound patient can perform 50 repetitions of Scapular Retraction (rowing) at 40 pounds of pull before fatigue, his Rhomboids are considered to be of normal strength.

  5.   Rhomboid and Middle Trapezius strengthening is the cornerstone of thoracic stabilization and functional lifting.

    a.   Therefore, the Shoulder Squeeze needs to be voluntarily contracted before any of the thoracic stabilization exercises or before any functional lifting activities such as work conditioning or work hardening.

    b.   Remember, as long as there is any upper back pain, the Rhomboids will NOT stabilize the thoracic spine due to reflex shut down.

E.   QUALITY of the neutral cervical stabilization exercises are paramount to the QUANTITY of exercises.

F.   As you progress a patient through the levels of stabilization, it is NOT necessary to continue the previous level's exercises as they are largely incorporated into the next level of exercise.

  1.   However, there may be times where multiple levels of spinal stabilization exercises need to be performed.

G.   The following Thoracic Stabilization Exercises are not all inclusive, however they represent exercises that will NOT create muscular imbalances in strength or flexibility.

  1.   These exercises also work all major muscle groups contributing to the balance of the thoracic spine.

  2.   Some of these exercises will be presented in the Cervical and/or Lumbar Spinal Stabilization sections as they contribute to spinal stability in those areas as well.

3. Recommended advanced exercises:
    a. There are two excellent resources for advanced spinal stabilization utilizing the Foam Roller and Swiss Ball apparatus by author Caroline Creager, PT and can be purchased at: OPTP Publications, 1-800-367-7393 or web site *www.optp.com*.

LEVEL 1 THORACIC STABILIZATION:

13-2 "Shoulder Squeeze"

Do not hold your breath.
Press/retract your shoulder blades together

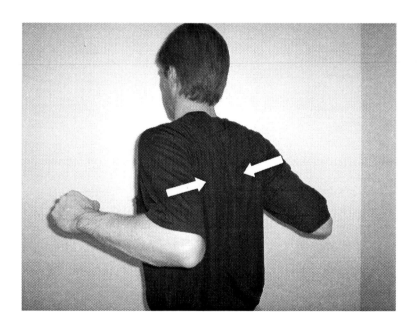

Hold >10 seconds as tolerated.
Relax and repeat 20 to 30 times as tolerated.

13-3 "External Rotation"

Do not hold your breath.
Perform the shoulder squeeze and hold the position.
Keep elbows in contact with the ribs.
Pull resistance band apart.

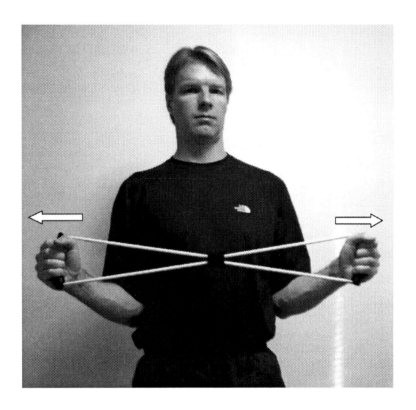

Hold 2 to 5 seconds as tolerated.
Relax and repeat up to 25 times as tolerated.

*Do not progress to level 2 unless symptoms are minimal.

LEVEL 2 THORACIC STABILIZATION

13-4 "Shoulder Extension"

Do not hold your breath.
Perform the shoulder squeeze and hold the position.
Keep the elbows extended and close to the body.
Pull resistance band backward.

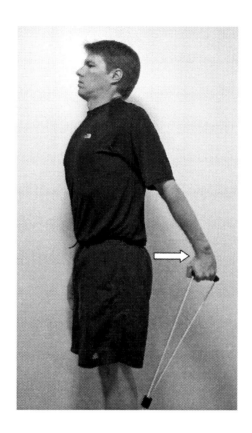

Hold 2 to 5 seconds.
Relax and repeat up to 25 times as tolerated.

13-5 "Saws"

Do not hold your breath.
Perform the shoulder squeeze and hold the position.
Pull the arm back and hold 2 to 5 seconds.

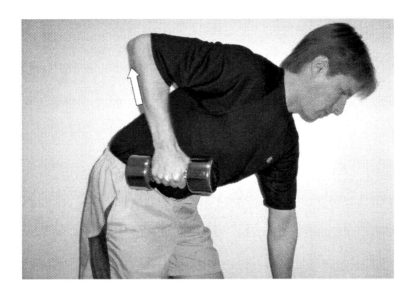

Relax and repeat up to 25 times as tolerated.

*May use resistance bands or dumbbell weights to increase resistance.
*Do not progress to Level 3 unless symptoms are minimal.

LEVEL 3 THORACIC STABILIZATION

13-6 "Scapular Protraction"

Do not hold your breath.
Lay supine.
Keep your elbows extended at all times.
Protract or round out the shoulder blades as you push toward the
    ceiling.

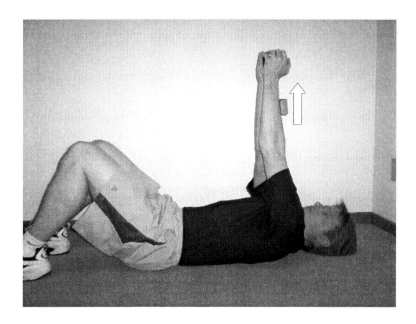

Hold 2 to 5 seconds.
Relax and repeat up to 25 times as tolerated.

*May use resistance bands or dumbbell weights to increase resistance.

13-7 "Overhead Isometric Extension"

Do not hold your breath.
Lay supine.
Keel your elbows extended at all times.
Push into the pillow and hold 2 to 5 seconds.

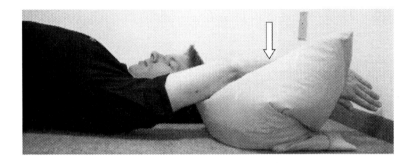

Relax and repeat up to 25 times as tolerated.

*Do not progress to Level 4 unless symptoms are minimal.

LEVEL 4 THORACIC STABILIZATION

13-8 "Prone Alternating Arm/Leg Extension"

Do not hold your breath.
Lay prone.
Perform the shoulder squeeze and hold.
Keep your elbows and knees extended.
Alternate right/left arm/leg lifts 1 to 3 inches off the mat

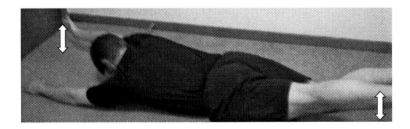

Hold 2 to 5 seconds.
Relax and repeat up to 25 times as tolerated.

13-9 "Superman"

Do not hold your breath.
Lay prone.
Perform the shoulder squeeze and hold.
Keep your elbows extended.
Lift both arms toward the ceiling 1 to 3 inches off the mat.

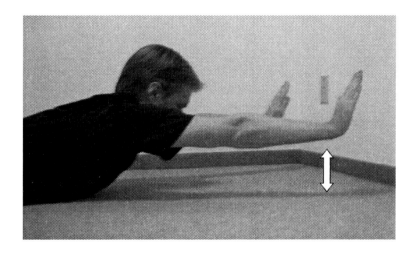

Hold 2 to 5 seconds.
Relax and repeat up to 25 times as tolerated.

*Do not progress to Level 5 unless symptoms are minimal.

Proven Therapeutic Exercise Techniques

LEVEL 5 THORACIC STABILIZATION

13-10 "Rocking Ball Forward/Back"

Do not hold your breath.
Perform the shoulder squeeze and hold the position.
Stabilize your wrists and put pressure on the Swiss ball.
Rock the ball forward and back 1 to 3 inches.

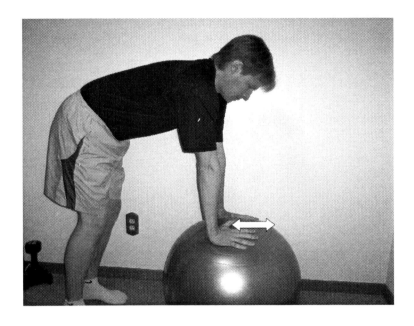

Alternate forward/backward rhythmical pattern up to 25 times as
   tolerated.

13-11 "Rocking Ball Side/Side"

Do not hold your breath.
Perform the shoulder squeeze and hold the position.
Stabilize your wrists and put pressure onto the Swiss ball.
Rock the ball side to side 1 to 3 inches.

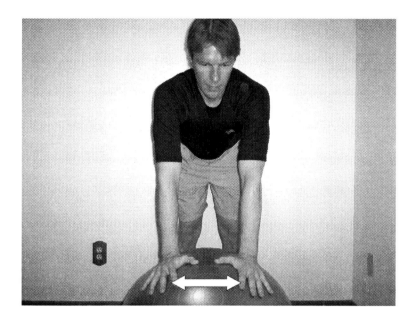

Alternate side/side rhythmical pattern up to 25 times as tolerated.

Chapter 14

PROVEN LUMBAR & SACRAL-ILIAC
SPINE EXERCISES

I. **Lumbar Spine Imbalances:** [4,19,34,47,48,51,53,61,63,64,70,71,72,77,83,
89,99,101,103,105,109,110,112,115,128,133,139,141]

A. How To Test Strength Imbalances in the Lumbar Spine:
1. Using a force dynamometer, the abdominal flexors
should be about $2/3$ as strong as the spinal extensors the
healthy patient population.
a. However, patients with low back pain generally do
not like the pressure of the dynamometer in their
back or stomach.
2. A better and more consistent way to test the balance
employs a strength and endurance combination test.
a. If you have access to an isotonic back extension
machine and trunk flexion machine, you may test
the patient by having them perform repetitive back
extension at approximately 50 percent of the patient s body weight until fatigued. Then test trunk
flexion at $2/3$ of the back extension weight until
fatigued.
i. For example, a 200 pound patient performed
35 repetitions of back extension at 100 pounds
of resistance with fatigue. Then the patient
performed 35 repetitions of trunk flexion at
60 pounds of resistance with fatigue. This example is a patient who has a normal muscle
balance anteriorly/posteriorly.
b. The problem with this method is the fact that if a
patient has back pain, spasms or a diagnosis that
becomes worse with repetitive flexion or extension
this test is skewed and invalid. This test is best for
the healthy back population.

216

3. Many patients will not tolerate either of the aforementioned tests if they have significant low back pain making testing difficult at best.
    a. However, one way that may be tolerated includes prone spinal extension in which the clavicle is held at a level approximately 1 inch above the mat table for a measured period of time.
    b. Then the trunk flexor strength/endurance is tested supine with the scapulae held approximately 1 inch above the mat table for a measured period of time.
        i. For example, if the patient holds spinal extension for 1 minute; he or she should be able to hold trunk flexion for about 40 seconds to be in balance.
B. Common Muscle Imbalances of the Lumbar Spine:
    1. Most often the spinal extensors (Erector Spinae group) is much stronger than the trunk flexors (Rectus Abdominis and Obliques) than the $1 : \frac{2}{3}$ ratio.
C. How To Test Muscle Flexibility Imbalances of the Lumbar Spine:
    1. Right to left imbalances of spinal flexibility are easily found with goniometric or inclinometric range of motion measurements.
        a. However, many flexibility issues involve the muscles that attach to the spine or pelvic girdle.
        b. Muscles commonly involved include the Iliopsoas, Rectus Femoris, Hamstrings, Piriformis, and Gluteals.
            i. The flexibility of these muscles are easily tested during an initial evaluation.
D. Common Flexibility Imbalances of the Lumbar Spine:
    1. I have found that the Piriformis and/or Iliopsoas muscles are commonly imbalanced and tight.
        a. The Piriformis muscle nearly always covers the sciatic nerve.
            i. Occasionally the sciatic nerve splits between portions of the Piriformis muscle.
        b. The Piriformis muscle originates on the Sacrum and inserts on the Greater Trochanter of the Femur.

i. The best way I have found to test the flexibility of the Piriformis is to have the patient lie supine and push the knee up and across the body to the opposite shoulder. (See Figure 14-1)

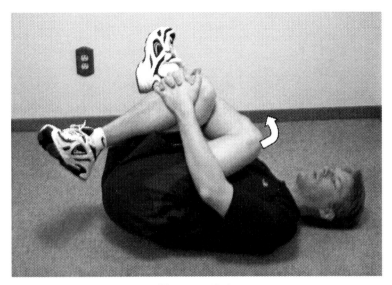

Figure 14-1

ii. The distance from the knee to the shoulder should be recorded. (Note: Some patients with excessive central obesity are difficult to measure accurately). The test is performed left and right. The distance from the shoulder left to right should not exceed 10% or an imbalance is indicated. Often the patient will also tell you which side felt tighter.

2. The Piriformis muscle if found tight will put excess pressure on the Sciatic Nerve causing the sciatic nerve to be pulled inferiorly (i.e., to the ground).

a. Simple anatomy will tell you that a tight Piriformis will also pull the individual lumbar nerve roots into the vertebral foramen possibly irritating the nerve and contributing to distal radicular signs and symptoms.

3. Another common sign of Piriformis tightness/entrapment of the Sciatic Nerve is excessive external rotation of the feet.
   a. The excess external foot rotation is also associated with central obesity or pregnancy.
4. The Iliopsoas and Quadrates Lumborum muscles provide additional resistance to spinal extension.
   a. The Iliopsoas originates on the Transverse Processes of T12-L5 and inserts on the Lesser Trochanter of the Femur.
   b. The Quadrates Lumborum originates on the Iliac Crest and L3-5 and inserts on Ribs #12 and Transverse Processes of L1-3.
      i. The best way I have found to test the flexibility of these muscles is to have the patient lie prone with a pillow under the knee. Gently push the heel toward the buttocks until tissue resistance is felt. Measure the distance between the heel and the buttocks and compare right to left. (See Figure 14-2)

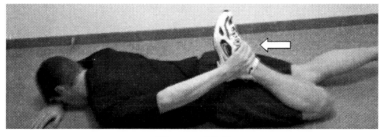

Figure 14-2

      ii. If these distances exceed 10 percent an imbalance is indicated. Again, the patient will often tell you which one feels tighter.
   b. It is important to note that the Iliopsoas and Quadrates Lumborum muscle imbalances can delay therapeutic goals and rehabilitative results especially in patients with Spondylolisthesis and Stenosis.

II. **Lumbar Spine Reflex Mechanisms:** [105]
   A. Largely based on the work of Richardson and Hodges. This spinal research group in Queensland, Australia has been sticking patients with electromyography (EMG) needles who suffer from low back pain for several years.
      1. The results of their studies have found that any legitimate low back pain will automatically shut down the Multifidus muscles of the lumbar spine.
      2. Remember, the Multifidus muscles are spinal stabilizers and occupy the space between the lumbar transverse processes.
         a. They contribute very little to lumbar extension, less than 5 percent.
         b. However, they contribute a significant amount to stabilizing the lumbar spine, (i.e., over 55 percent).
   B. What happens when the Multifidus muscles shut down?
      1. The Erector Spinae group of muscles now have 2 jobs:
         a. They are responsible for moving the lumbar spine, primarily for extension.
         b. And now they must also try and stabilize the lumbar spine.
            i. This over stresses the Erector Spinae muscles and causes pain, spasms, and fatigue.
   C. The Australian research group has shown that in order to rehabilitate the Multifidus muscles we must employ a reflex mechanism.
      1. A reflex exists between the Transversus Abdominis muscle contraction and the Multifidus muscles. In short, when the Transversus Abdominis muscle is contracted in the Belly Lift exercise, the Multifidus muscles automatically (or reflexively) contract.
      2. The Belly Lift is the key and cornerstone to lumbar stabilization.
         a. Belly Lift exercises should be performed prior to any other lumbar strengthening exercises. (See Figure 14-3)

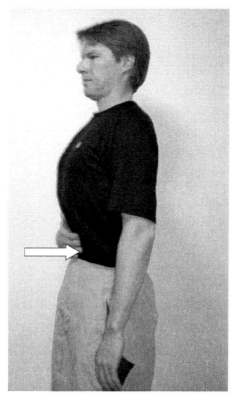

Figure 14-3

3. Oddly enough, the researchers concluded that the
    Transversus Abdominis is also a spinal stabilizer.
    a. This muscle only contributes about 5 percent to the
        flexion of the trunk (i.e., during a sit up or abdomi-
        nal crunch).
    b. However, the relationship between the Transversus
        Abdominis and Multifidus is important because
        they are responsible for the majority of lumbar sta-
        bility and successful spinal rehabilitation.
D. In patients without low back pain, EMG studies show that
    the Transversus Abdominis fires just before the Multifidus
    when lifting.
    1. This is precisely why we concentrate on isolating the
        Transversus Abdominis in order to strengthen the
        Multifidus.

III. **Lumbar Spine Nerve Extensibility:** [113]
   A.   Duane Saunders is a pioneer in developing eclectic spinal evaluations and treatment approaches. According to his research and works, nerve extensibility is the most often overlooked evaluative technique in the lumbar spine.
   B.   The spinal canal is surrounded by a tough plastic like substance called, "Dura."
      1.   It provides additional protection to the spinal cord.
      2.   The "Dural Sleeve" as it is often referred to slides superiorly and inferiorly a few millimeters with spinal movements, especially flexion.
   C.   As many spinal injuries heal, the healing process lays down collagen and elastin fibers to scar or reinforce the injured area.
      1.   Unfortunately some of this scarring lays down spider web like fibers attaching the Dural Sleeve to the spinal vertebrae.
      2.   This reduces the mobility of the Dura, and often entraps or limits the nerve root migration with spinal movements thus causing pain.
   D.   How to Test for Lower Limb Tissue Tension/Dural Extensibility:
      1.   This test must be performed very carefully, and it is NOT recommended for patients with HNP diagnoses.
      2.   Sit the patient and allow them to flex the head and neck, round out the thoracic spine, and flex the lumbar spine. The SLOWLY raise one foot to extend the lower leg. Have the patient SLOWLY dorsiflex the foot. Pain or discomfort in the sciatic distribution along the hamstring is normal. However, pain or discomfort deep within the spinal canal, usually lumbar or thoracic indicates problems with dural extensibility. Test left, then right legs separately. (See Figure 14-4)

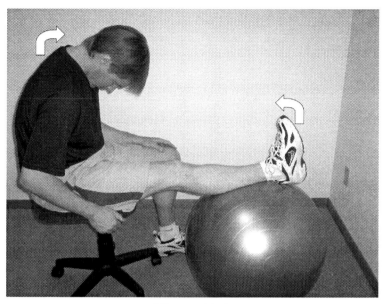

Figure 14-4

E. How To Improve Dural Extensibility:
   1. Dural Extensibility is improved the same way you
       tested for it. Have the patient hold each stretch 15 to
       20 seconds and repeat 3 to 5 times. As the symptoms
       improve, you may have them alternately dorsiflex
       and plantarflex the foot often referred to as "Neural
       Flossing."
   2. This is NOT difficult to have patients do independently
       if properly trained and demonstrative.

IV. **Commonly Overlooked Lumbar & Sacral Iliac Spine Conditions:** 4,19,34,47,48,51,53,61,63,64,70,71,72,77,83,89,99,101,103,105,109,110,112, 115,128,133,139,141

   A. Muscle imbalances in the lumbar spine, trunk and lower extremities are very common with Ilial-Sacral and Sacral-Ilial pathologies.
       1. While not a text on differential diagnosis, the following
           are commonly overlooked in the process of properly
           evaluating and diagnosing a patient:
           a. If low back pain does NOT resolve with Neutral
               Lumbar Stabilization exercises, it is often due
               to one or more of the following pathologies as
               described:

      i.   Abnormal movement in the pelvic girdle is suspected to alter the Ilia and cause pain symptoms to be reported on the opposite side of the hypomobility.

     ii.   Anterior pelvic tilt is often associated with pelvic inflare and excess hip internal rotation or limited hip external rotation.

   iii.   Posterior pelvic tilt is often associated with pelvic outflare and excess hip external rotation or limited hip internal rotation.

B.   Spinal range of motion is limited if:
1. Forward bending >20 cm finger tip to floor.
2. Side bending >10 cm finger tip to floor.
3. Rotation <45 degrees and/or asymmetrical >10 degrees compared to opposite side.[18]

C.   If spinal range of motion is limited it often indicates Facet Subluxations or Facet Blocks as follows:
1. Active Range of Motion (AROM) deviates toward the involved side with forward bending.
2. Pain occurs with side bending away from involved side.
3. Pain occurs with rotation toward involved side.

D.   Herniated Nucleus Pulposus (HNP) diagnosis is suspected if:
1. Pain is worse in the morning than in the evening.
2. Symptoms become better with activity.
3. Back pain is worse than leg pain.
4. Pain becomes worse with sitting, sneezing and coughing.

E.   Prolapsed Disc diagnosis is suspected if:
1. Pain is worse in evening than in the morning.
2. Symptoms become worse with activity.
3. Leg pain is worse than back pain.
4. Pain becomes worse with standing or walking, but sneezing and coughing do not affect it.

F.   Ilial-Sacral Dysfunctions such as anterior or posterior rotated Innominates, up slipped or down slipped Innominates and Ilial inflares or outflares are suspected if:
1. Pain becomes worse with walking.
2. Sitting and sleeping do not cause pain.
3. Stiffness is greater in the morning.
4. Sit to stand transfers are painful.
5. Sidebending is painful.

6. Active hip extension from full flexion pops at 50 to 70 degrees of hip flexion.

G. Sacral-Iliac Dysfunctions such as forward or backward torsions and flexed or extended Sacrums have all of the symptoms of Ilial-Sacral Dysfunctions with the common presentation of a stiff legged gait.

V. **Neutral Lumbar Spine Stabilization Exercises:**[4,19,34,47, 48,51,53,61,63,64,70,71,72,77,83,89,99,101,103,105,109,110,112,115,128,133,139,141]

A. Lumbar stabilization employs the concept of a neutral spine.
1. Make sure the neutral lumbar spine is maintained for all exercises.
2. Lumbar stabilization follows a defined sequence from easy to hard.
3. Most patients begin with 5 to 10 exercises, and progress 5 repetitions per week to a maximum of 25 repetitions for each exercise.
4. We do not recommend any continuous repetitions over 25 repetitions because of the risk of overuse injury or tendonitis.

B. Stretches for muscle imbalances or nerve imbalances should be performed before lumbar stabilization to minimize inadvertent spinal stresses.
1. Exercises for muscle weakness imbalances should also be performed before lumbar stabilization to minimize inadvertent spinal stresses.

C. Modalities such as superficial heat, cold, ultrasound, electrical stimulation and cervical traction may be performed before or after lumbar stabilization exercises depending on the clinician's purpose, and of course as long as they are NOT contraindicated.

D. Lumbar Stabilization exercises are appropriate for ALL lumbar spine pathologies and diagnoses during some course of their healing stage. However, there are two types of specialty exercises that may be utilized independently or in combination (BEFORE or AFTER) lumbar stabilization exercises (depending on the clinician's purpose):
1. If the clinician s purpose is to minimize pain before performing Neutral Lumbar Stabilization, he/she should perform the McKenzie or Williams exercises before the Lumbar Stabilization. This will minimize discomfort

during stabilization exercises and minimize the pain reflex shut down of the Multifidus muscles.

2. However, if the clinician s purpose is to maximize anterior disc migration with McKenzie Extension, or to maximize spinal columnar and foraminal space with Williams Flexion, these types of exercises would be better performed after completing Neutral Lumbar Stabilization.

3. McKenzie Extension exercises are appropriate for the following spinal diagnoses: HNP; Sprain/Strains, Retrolisthesis.

    a. Examples of McKenzie Extension exercises include Prone Press Ups, and Alternate Arm/Leg Lifts.

4. Williams Flexion exercises are appropriate for the following spinal diagnoses: Stenosis, Spondylolysis, Spondylolisthesis.

    a. Examples of Williams Flexion exercises include Double Knee to Chest, and Abdominal Crunches.

E. Level 1 Lumbar Stabilization is the cornerstone of all advanced levels of stabilization.

1. The Transversus Abdominis exercise (commonly referred to as the "Belly Lift") should be performed before initiating any level 2 to 5 exercise and held throughout the exercise.

2. Most lumbar stabilization exercises should be held 2 to 5 seconds, and repeated up to 25 repetitions as long as the neutral spine is NOT compromised.

3. The Transversus Abdominis is contracted by the following command:

    a. "Lift your belly button toward your spine."

    b. Do not hold your breath, or you are utilizing the Diaphragm muscle to assist with this task. (See Figure 14-3)

4. Positions To Perform Belly Lifts:

    a. ALL positions: prone, four point, tall kneeling, standing, and sitting are appropriate.

    b. Standing or Four point are the preferred positions to initially instruct patients on the exercise because it is easiest to relax the Erector Spinae muscles.

3. How long do you hold the Belly Lift contraction?

    a. At least 10 seconds, for 20 to 30 repetitions.

        i. Ten seconds of contraction generally allows patients enough time to complete a brief lifting task in which the Multifidus will automatically be contracted thus maximizing stability to the lumbar spine and reducing the possibility of injury.

4. How do you know when the Transversus Abdominis is of normal strength?

    a. Based on empirical data I have collected on thousands of patients with low back pain, I have found the best way to establish a baseline and follow-up measurement is to have the patient lay prone with a folded up blood pressure cuff under the belly button.

        i. Pump the cuff up to 50 mmHG. Instruct the patient to relax the belly and breathe normally. Then instruct the patient to lift the belly button toward the spine and record the blood pressure cuff measurement upon initial instruction, then upon discharge or re-evaluation to chart progress. While lifting the belly button the patient needs to continue to breathe normally.

       ii. I have found that most baseline measures in patients with low back pain ranges from a 2-4 mmHG drop in pressure. This is particularly true among any patient with any diagnosis, obese or thin, young or old.

      iii. I have found that in patients with no back pain, or in those who have resolved their back pain that the pressure in the cuff drops 10 mmHG. Again, this is particularly true among any patient young or old, obese or thin.

      iv. This is empirical data that I have measured and recorded since 1995 and should be useful to you in writing goals, (i.e., "Increase Transversus Abdominis strength of contraction to 10 mmHG by 6 weeks in order to decrease pain and spasms to resume normal work duties of lifting up to 20 pounds on a "frequent" basis without exacerbation of symptoms.")

5. The Belly Lift is the cornerstone of lumbar stabilization and functional lifting.
   a. It needs to be voluntarily contracted before any of the lumbar stabilization exercises or before any functional lifting activities such as work conditioning or work hardening.
   b. Remember, as long as there is any low back pain, the Multifidus will not stabilize the lumbar spine without a voluntary Transversus Abdominis contraction.

F. Another part of Level 1 Lumbar Stabilization is voluntary contraction of the Multifidus muscles.
   1. Remember, these muscles are automatically shut down in patients with back pain.
   2. While the Belly Lift exercise voluntarily contracts the Transversus Abdominis, it also reflexively contracts the Multifidus.
   3. However, voluntary contraction of the Mutifidus muscle is prerequisite for total rehabilitation and re-training of the muscle function:
   4. The Multifidus is contracted by the following command, "Pull your hip up into the socket." Do NOT arch your back when performing this exercise. (See Figure 14-5)
      a. The Hip Hiking exercise involves a very small movement, less than one inch of movement.
      b. This is best performed in the prone position with the clinician's fingers palpating between the transverse processes of the lumbar spine.
         i. Make sure that the Erector Spinae muscles do NOT contract.
   5. How long do you hold the Multifidus contraction?
      a. At least 10 seconds, for 20 to 30 repetitions.
         i. Ten seconds of contraction generally allows patients enough time to complete a brief lifting task thus maximizing stability to the lumbar spine and reducing the possibility of injury.

6. How do you know when the Multifidus is of normal strength?
   a. I have not found consistent empirical or scientific data to isolate this muscle which is why I use the Transverse Abdominis for testing, because it is representative of the Multifidus strength.
   b. Remember the Transversus Abdominis and Multifidus work together via a reflex.
      i. If the Transversus Abdominis is contracted, the Multifidus automatically (i.e., reflexively) contracts.

E. QUALITY of the neutral lumbar stabilization exercises are paramount to the QUANTITY of exercises.

F. As you progress a patient through the levels of stabilization, it is NOT necessary to continue the previous level's exercises as they are largely incorporated into the next level of exercise.
   1. However, there may be times where multiple levels of spinal stabilization exercises need to be performed.

G. The following Lumbar Stabilization Exercises are not all inclusive, however they represent exercises that will NOT create muscular imbalances in strength or flexibility.
   1. These exercises also work all major muscle groups contributing to the stability of the lumbar spine.
   2. There is an old saying in rehabilitation that goes, "Proximal Stability for Distal Mobility." Many of the lumbar stabilization exercises involve working the abdominal and core trunk muscles. The stronger the core, the less stress that will occur in the lumbar spine as well as the lower extremities.
   3. Recommended advanced exercises:
      a. There are two excellent resources for advanced spinal stabilization utilizing the Foam Roller and Swiss Ball apparatus by author Caroline Creager, PT and can be purchased at: OPTP Publications, 1-800-367-7393 or web site *www.optp.com*.

LEVEL 1 LUMBAR STABILIZATION:

14-3 "Belly Lift"

Do not hold your breath.
Lift your belly button toward your spine.
(Suck in your stomach)

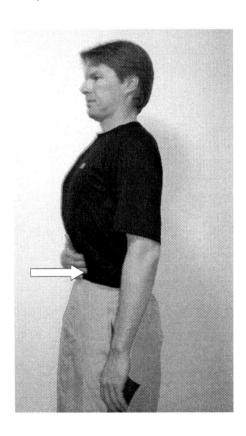

Hold >10 seconds as tolerated.
Relax and repeat 20 to 30 times as tolerated.

14-5 "Multifidus Exercise"

Do not hold your breath.
Gently pull your hip (right then left) up into the socket
(Hike your hip up)

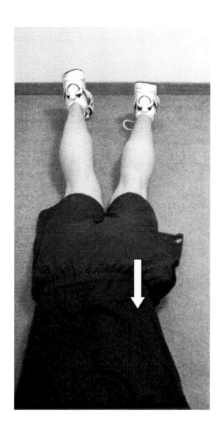

Hold 2 to 5 seconds as tolerated.
Relax and repeat up to 25 times as tolerated.

*Do not progress to level 2 unless symptoms are minimal.

LEVEL 2 LUMBAR STABILIZATION

14-6 "Alternating Supine Leg Kicks"

Do not hold your breath.
Perform the belly lift and hold.
Slowly kick one leg out and back.
Do NOT raise the leg above the level of the opposite knee.
Alternate legs right and left.

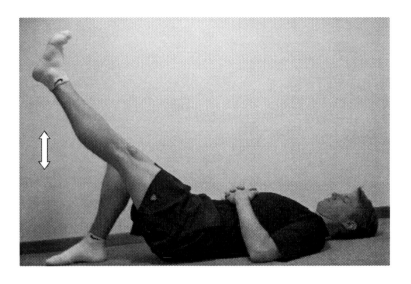

Hold 2 to 5 seconds.
Relax and repeat up to 25 times as tolerated.

14-7 "Alternating Supine Arm/Leg Kicks"

Do not hold your breath.
Perform the belly lift and hold.
Bring opposite hand and knee together, then extend apart.
Alternate right, then left.

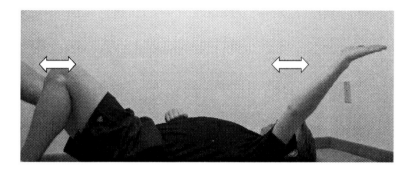

Hold 2 to 5 seconds.
Relax and repeat up to 25 times as tolerated.

*Do not progress to Level 3 unless symptoms are minimal.

LEVEL 3 LUMBAR STABILIZATION

14-8 "Sitting Knee Lifts"

Do not hold your breath.
Perform the belly lift and hold.
Slowly raise one knee up and lower.
Alternate knee lifts right, then left.

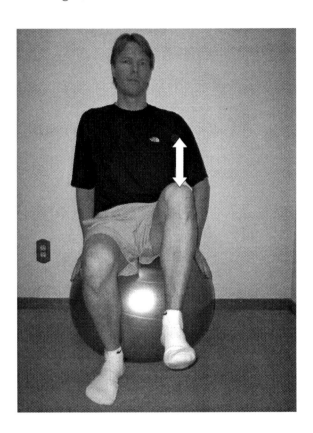

Hold 2 to 5 seconds.
Relax and repeat up to 25 times as tolerated.

*May use resistance bands or sandbag weights to increase resistance.

14-9 "Alternate Arm/Leg Kicks Sitting"

Do not hold your breath.
Perform the belly lift and hold.
Bring opposite hand and knee together, then extend apart.
Alternate right, then left.

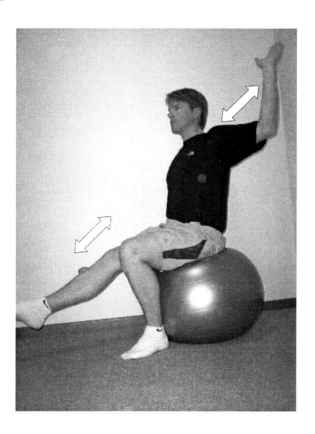

Hold 2 to 5 seconds.
Relax and repeat up to 25 times as tolerated.
Do not progress to Level 4 unless symptoms are minimal.

LEVEL 4 LUMBAR STABILIZATION

14-10 "4 Point Leg Kicks"

Do not hold your breath.
Perform the Belly Lift and hold.
Slowly extend your leg outward.
Do NOT raise the leg above the level of the hip.
Alternate right, then left.

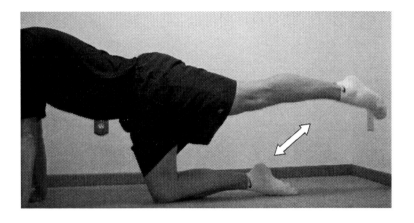

Hold 2 to 5 seconds.
Relax and repeat up to 25 times as tolerated.

14-11 "4 Point Alternating Arm/Leg Kicks"

Do not hold your breath.
Perform the Belly Lift and hold.
Bring opposite hand and knee together, then extend apart.
Alternate right, then left.

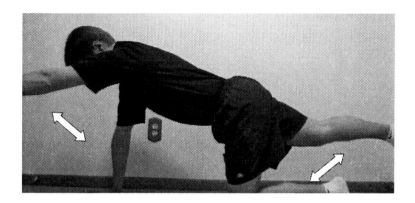

Hold 2 to 5 seconds.
Relax and repeat up to 25 times as tolerated.

*Do not progress to Level 5 unless symptoms are minimal.

LEVEL 5 LUMBAR STABILIZATION

14-12 "Bridging"

Do not hold your breath.
Perform the Belly Lift and hold.
Squeeze your buttocks together and lift 1 to 3 inches, then lower.

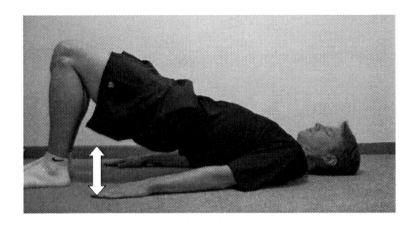

Hold 2 to 5 seconds.
Relax and repeat up to 25 times as tolerated.

14-13 "Bridging Leg Kicks"

Do not hold your breath.
Perform the Belly Lift and hold.
Hold the Bridging position with your buttocks off the floor 1 to 3 inches.
Slowly extend one leg outward and return.
Alternate right, then left.

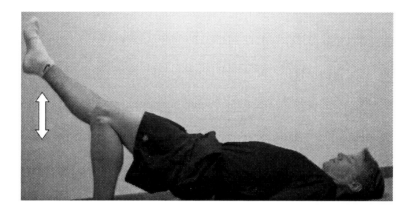

Hold 2 to 5 seconds.
Relax and repeat up to 25 times as tolerated.

14-14 "Cowboy"

Do not hold your breath.
Perform the Belly Lift and hold.
Maintain upright posture.
Bring opposite hand and knee together, then extend apart.
Alternate right, then left.

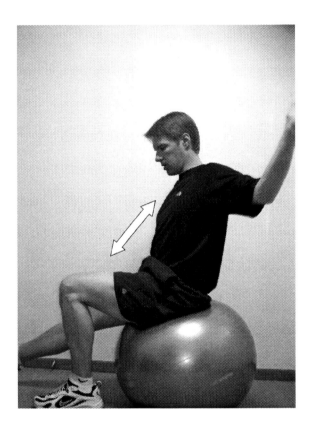

Alternate right/left rhythmical pattern up to 25 times as tolerated.

14-15 "Sit Backs"

Do not hold your breath.
Perform the Belly Lift and hold.
Roll back and forth on the ball.
The hips and knees will flex/extend.
Keep the spine stable.

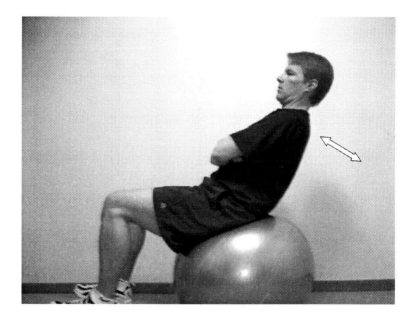

Hold 2 to 5 seconds.
Relax and repeat up to 25 times as tolerated.

14-16 "Walk Outs"

Do not hold your breath.
Perform the Belly Lift and hold.
Walk yourself out and back with your arms.
Do NOT allow the spine to arch.

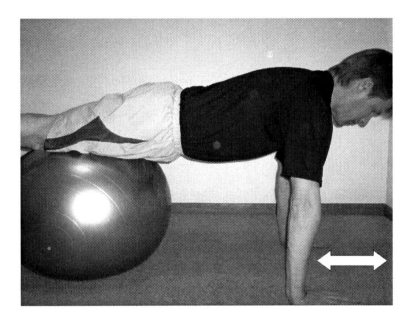

Move forward and backward in a rhythmical pattern up to 25 times as
tolerated.

PROVEN WILLIAMS FLEXION EXERCISES

14-17 "Double Knee To Chest"

Do not hold your breath.
Pull both knees up to the chest and hold.

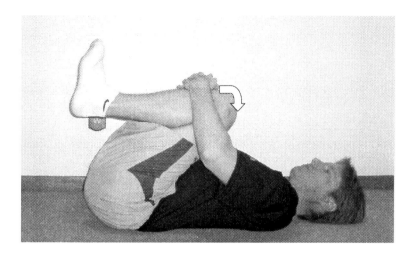

Hold 2 to 5 seconds.
Relax and repeat up to 25 times as tolerated.

14-18 "Abdominal Crunches"

Do not hold your breath.
Slowly curl the shoulders off the floor 1 to 3 inches.

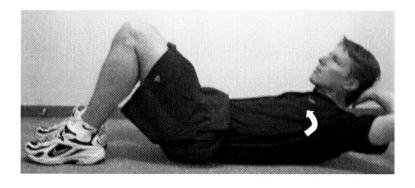

Hold 2 to 5 seconds.
Relax and repeat up to 25 times as tolerated.

PROVEN MCKENZIE EXTENSION EXERCISES

14-19 "Prone Press Ups"

Do not hold your breath.
Relax the back muscles and just use your arms.
Push your body up with your arms, leaving your pelvis flat on the floor.

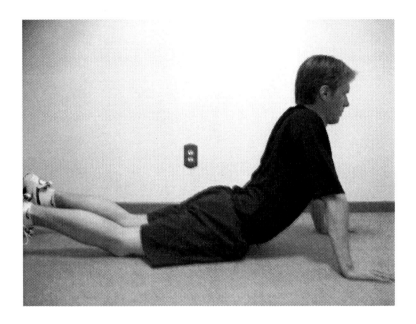

Hold 2 to 5 seconds.
Relax and repeat up to 25 times as tolerated.

14-20 "Prone Alternate Arm/Leg Lifts"

Do not hold your breath.
Alternately extend one arm and the opposite leg as high as possible.

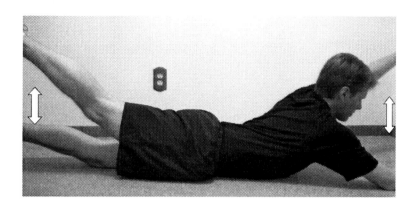

Hold 2 to 5 seconds.
Relax and repeat up to 25 times as tolerated.

Part 5

SPECIAL CONSIDERATIONS – PROVEN TECHNIQUES

Chapter 15

OSTEOARTHRITIS–PROVEN TECHNIQUES

I. **Preparations:**
A. ALL of the contraindications, precautions, indications, goals/and effects listed in Chapter 2 apply to the proven exercise techniques in this chapter.

II. **Osteoarthritis Background:**[34,41,47,50,63,64,93,123,131]
A. Osteoarthritis is a non-inflammatory degenerative condition involving the hyaline cartilage and subchondral bone affecting nearly 20 million people in the United States.
B. As the disease process progresses cartilage and bone begin to erode away.
C. Females and males are equally affected by Osteoarthritis.
D. Osteoarthritis is most common in the weight bearing joints of the hip, knee and back.
E. However, the Proximal Interphalangeal and Distal Interphalangeal joints of the fingers are also commonly affected by Osteoarthritis.
F. Heberden's nodes on the Distal Interphalangeal joints of the fingers are telltale signs of Osteoarthritis.
G. Symptoms are normally the worst in the morning and get better as the day progresses. Therefore, exercise in the afternoon is preferred in patients with Osteoarthritis.
H. The top 7 proven treatment recommendations by the National Institute of Arthritis include:
1. Medications including acetaminophen and prescription medications.
2. Cryotherapy, heat therapy and/or analgesic modalities.
3. Joint protection utilizing splints, braces and wraps.
4. Massage therapy.
5. Weight reduction and special diets including vitamin and mineral supplements.

      6.   Surgery in the advanced stages to provide pain relief and improve function.

      7.   Therapeutic exercise that includes swimming, walking, low-impact aerobic exercise and specific range of motion exercises prescribed by a clinician.

  I.   It is important to respect the pain associated with Osteoarthritis:

      1.   Activities and therapeutic exercise will cause discomfort, but if it lasts more than one to two hours, cut back activities and exercise 50 percent for the next day.

      2.   If the same result occurs the next day, cut the activities another 50 percent until the discomfort lasts only one to two hours. Only then can you begin to increase activity.

III. **Proven Osteoarthritis Therapeutic Exercises:**[34,41,47,50,63,64,93,123,131]

  A.   While there are hundreds of researchers who have tested the efficacy of various exercises on Osteoarthritis, no cohort retains exclusive acknowledgement for the following eclectic recommendations which are based on the most common areas affected, also known as the "3 × 10" exercises:

      1.   Ten minutes of low impact aerobic exercise such as walking, bicycling or elliptical gliding comprise phase 1.

      2.   Ten repetitions performed three times for strengthening exercise comprise phase 2.

      3.   Ten minutes of gentle stretching exercises comprise phase 3.

PHASE 1

15-1 "10 Minutes Low Impact Aerobic Exercise"

Perform 10 minutes of low impact aerobic exercise such as walking, bicycling or elliptical gliding.
Elliptical gliding is shown here.

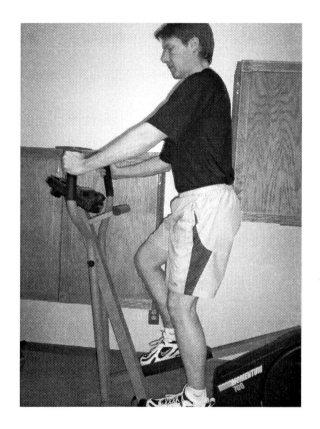

PHASE 2

15-2 "Rowing"

Do NOT hold your breath.
Start from an extended arm position.
Pull backward using the shoulder blades first, then the arms.

*Do NOT allow your wrists back beyond the vertical plane of the hip

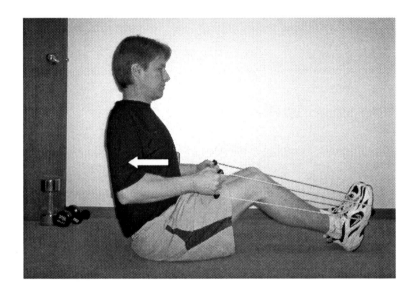

Hold 2 to 5 seconds.
Relax and repeat up to 10 times in 3 sets of exercise as tolerated.

15-3 "Bridging"

Do not hold your breath.
Squeeze your buttocks together and lift 1 to 3 inches, then lower.

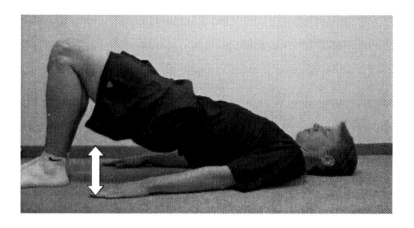

Hold 2 to 5 seconds.
Relax and repeat up to 10 times in 3 sets of exercise as tolerated.

15-4 "Mini Wall Slides"

Do NOT hold your breath.
Lean up against a wall.
Slide down the wall about 2 to 4 inches.

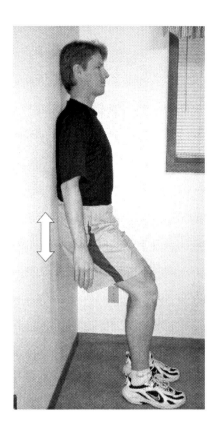

Hold for 2 to 5 seconds.
Then raise up and repeat up to 10 times in 3 sets of exercise as
   tolerated.

*NEVER squat down below a 75 degree bend at the knee.

PHASE 3

15-5 "Piriformis Stretch"

Do not hold your breath.
Lay supine and cross the legs.

*Sitting upright and crossing the legs is an acceptable position substitute for those who cannot lay supine or who may have excess central obesity.

Pull the knee that is on top of the other up and across the body to the opposite shoulder.

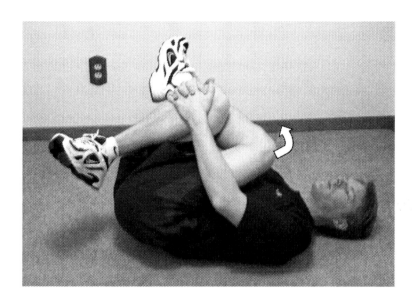

Hold 15 to 30 seconds as tolerated.
Relax and repeat 3 to 5 times as tolerated.

15-6 "Hamstring Stretch"

Do not hold your breath.
Gently lean forward, keeping your back straight and reach for your
    toes.
Perform on each leg independently.

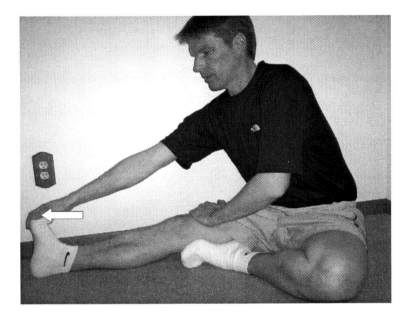

Hold 15 to 30 seconds as tolerated.
Relax and repeat 3 to 5 times as tolerated.

15-7 "Calf Stretch"

Do not hold your breath.
Keep your knees straight and allow your heels to drop stretching the
  calf muscles.

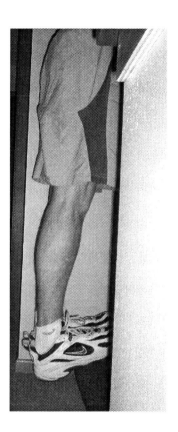

Hold 15 to 30 seconds as tolerated.
Relax and repeat 3 to 5 times as tolerated.

15-8 "High Corner Stretch"

Do not hold your breath.
Place one arm flat on each wall in the corner of a room.
Lean into the wall until you feel a modest stretch in the chest and arms.

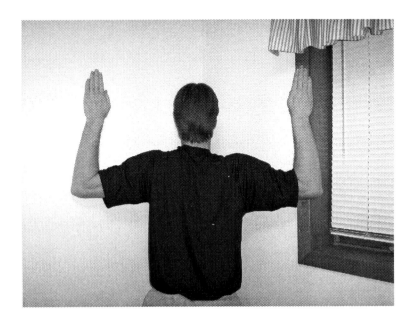

Hold the stretch 15 to 30 seconds as tolerated.
Relax and repeat 3 to 5 times as tolerated.

15-9 "Spinal Stretch"

Do not hold your breath.

Lay supine if able and press your neck down flat, keeping your shoulders back and press your lower back flat into the floor.

*Essentially you want to flatten the entire spine and elongate it.

*Performing this standing against a wall is a suitable substitute if unable to assume the supine position.

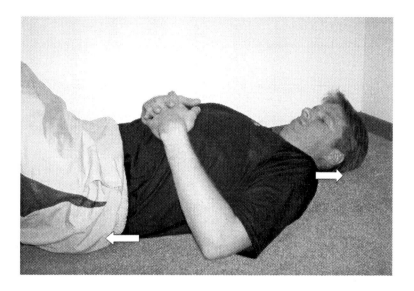

Hold 15 to 30 seconds as tolerated.

Relax and repeat 3 to 5 times as tolerated.

Chapter 16

RHEUMATOID ARTHRITIS–
PROVEN TECHNIQUES

I. **Preparations:**
    A. ALL of the contraindications, precautions, indications, goals/and effects listed in Chapter 2 apply to the proven exercise techniques in this chapter.

II. **Rheumatoid Arthritis Background:**[34,41,47,50,63,64,93,121,123]
    A. Rheumatoid arthritis is an inflammatory condition involving the synovial membrane in joint capsules affecting nearly 2.1 million people in the United States.
    B. As the disease process progresses joint, bone, capsule and ligaments begin to erode away.
    C. Females are 2 to 3 times more likely to have Rheumatoid arthritis than males.
    D. Rheumatoid arthritis is most common in the peripheral joints like the elbow, wrist, fingers, ankles and toes.
    E. Muscle contractures and an ulnar drift of the fingers are tell-tale signs of Rheumatoid arthritis.
    F. A simple blood test is the most conclusive and easiest way to diagnose Rheumatoid arthritis.
    G. Symptoms are normally the worst in the evening after much activity. Therefore, exercise in the morning is preferred in patients with Rheumatoid arthritis.
    H. The top 7 proven treatment recommendations by the National Institute of Arthritis include:
        1. Medications including non-steroidal anti-inflammatory drugs and prescription medications.
        2. Cryotherapy and other anti-inflammatory or analgesic modalities.
        3. Joint protection utilizing splints, braces and wraps.
        4. Massage therapy.

     5. Weight reduction and special diets including vitamin and mineral supplements.

     6. Surgery in the advanced stages to provide pain relief and improve function.

     7. Therapeutic exercise that includes swimming, walking, low-impact aerobic exercise and specific range of motion exercises prescribed by a clinician.

I. It is important to respect the pain associated with Rheumatoid arthritis:

     1. Activities and therapeutic exercise will cause discomfort, but if it lasts more than one to two hours, cut back activities and exercise 50 percent for the next day.

     2. If the same result occurs the next day, cut the activities another 50 percent until the discomfort lasts only one to two hours. Only then can you begin to increase activity.

III. **Proven Rheumatoid Arthritis Therapeutic Exercises:** [34, 41,47,50,63,64,93,121,123]

    A. While there are hundreds of researchers who have tested the efficacy of various exercises on Rheumatoid arthritis, no cohort retains exclusive acknowledgement for the following eclectic recommendations which are based on the most common areas affected, also known as the "5 × 25" exercises:

16-1 "Radial Drift Finger Exercises"

Do NOT hold your breath.

Hold all the fingers together and move them simultaneously toward the thumb.

The amount of movement will be small and you may need to assist with the other hand.

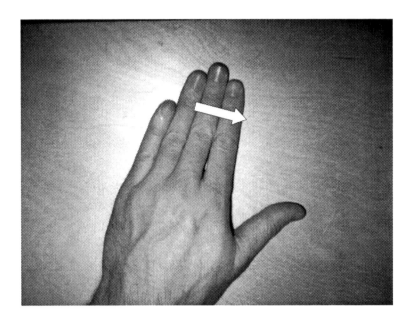

Hold for 2 to 5 seconds.

Relax and repeat up to 25 times as tolerated.

16-2 "Corkscrews"

Do not hold your breath.
Begin with the elbow extended forearm pronated, holding a dumbbell weight.
Bend your elbow and simultaneously supinated the forearm.

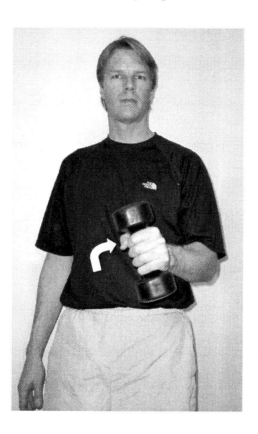

Hold 2 to 5 seconds.
Relax and repeat up to 25 times as tolerated.

16-3 "Reverse Corkscrews"

Do not hold your breath.
Begin with the elbow extended forearm supinated, holding a dumbbell
    weight.
Bend your elbow and simultaneously pronate the forearm.

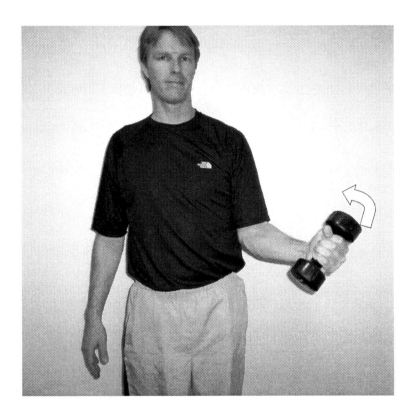

Hold 2 to 5 seconds.
Relax and repeat up to 25 times as tolerated.

16-4 "Mini Wall Slides"

Do NOT hold your breath.
Lean up against a wall.
Slide down the wall about 2 to 4 inches.

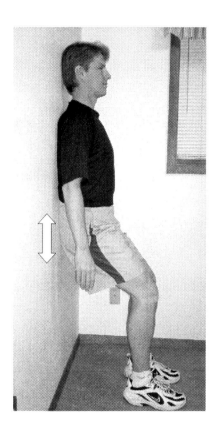

Hold for 2 to 5 seconds.
Relax and repeat up to 25 times as tolerated.

16-5 "Ankle Pumps"

Do NOT hold your breath/
Maximally dorsiflex and plantarflex your foot.

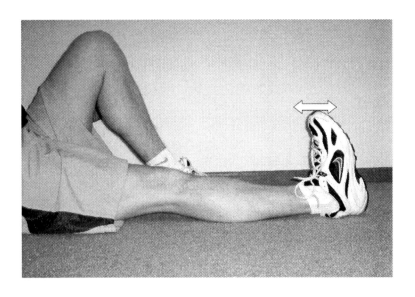

Hold 2 to 5 seconds.
Relax and repeat up to 25 times as tolerated.

Chapter 17

VESTIBULAR DYSFUNCTION–
PROVEN TECHNIQUES

I. **Preparations:**
    A. ALL of the contraindications, precautions, indications, goals/and effects listed in Chapter 2 apply to the proven exercise techniques in this chapter.

II. **Vestibular Dysfunction Background:** [34,63,64,115,123,137]
    A. Vestibular dysfunction often results in vertigo/dizziness in a commonly overlooked condition called, "Benign Paroxysmal Positional Vertigo" or (BPPV).
    B. BPPV is caused by otoconia which consist of small calcium carbonate crystals in the utricle of the inner ear.
    C. The otoconia can become dislodged and free float in the inner ear vestibular canal system due to head injury, infection and/or degeneration associated with advanced age.
    D. When the otoconia become dislodged from the cilia, they are moved with patient positions and stimulate vestibular canal cilia thus giving the brain the improper signal of movement. Dizziness, vertigo and often nausea are the result.
    E. Nearly 50 percent of all cases of vertigo are related to BPPV.
    F. BPPV is NOT the same as Meniere's disease which is characterized by hearing loss and true rotary vertigo and tinnitus.
        1. The proven techniques outlined in this chapter do not improve Meniere's disease, unless of course BPPV is an accompanying diagnosis.

III. **Proven Vestibular Dysfunction Therapeutic Exercises:**
    [34,63,64,115,123,137]

    A. Based on the research of Epley, Semont, Brandt and Daroff, the following sequential exercises, often referred to as

267

"Canalith Repositioning," succeed in 80 to 95 percent of all BPPV cases and are as follows:

17-1 "Step One"

Do not hold your breath.

Sit upright and look straight ahead.

It is important to hold the position for at least 30 seconds or until nystagmus stops before moving to step two.

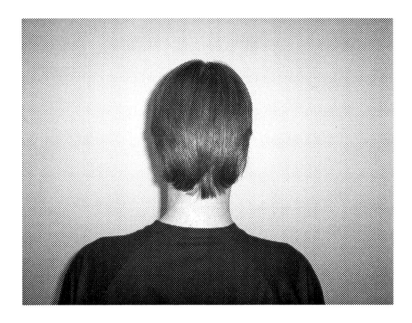

17-2 "Step Two"

Do not hold your breath.
Lay supine and turn your head 45 degrees to the right.
Keep your eyes focused on an object straight ahead.
It is important to hold the position for at least 30 seconds or until nystagmus stops before moving to step three.

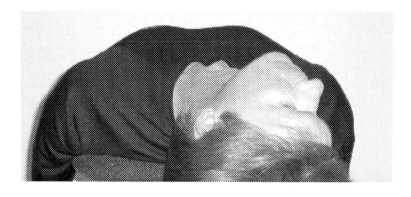

17-3 "Step Three"

Do not hold your breath.
Stay on your back and slowly turn your head 45 degrees to the left.
Keep your eyes focused on an object straight ahead.
It is important to hold the position for at least 30 seconds or until nystagmus stops before moving to step four.

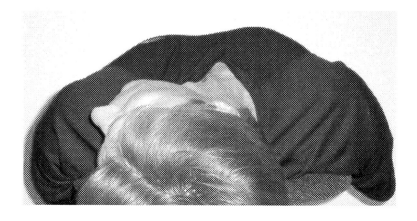

17-4 "Step Four"

Do not hold your breath.
Keep your head turned at 45 degrees to the left while rolling onto your
    left side.
Keep your eyes focused on an object straight ahead.
It is important to hold the position for at least 30 seconds or until nys-
    tagmus stops before moving to step five.

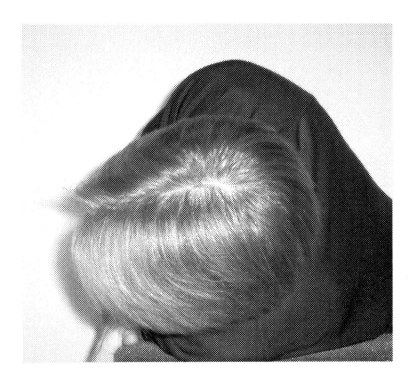

17-5 "Step Five"

Do not hold your breath.

Keep your head turned at 45 degrees to the left while slowly sitting upright.

Keep your eyes focused on an object straight ahead.

It is important to hold the position for at least 30 seconds or until nystagmus stops before moving to step six.

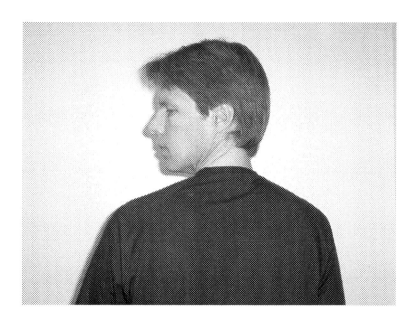

"Step Six"

Do not hold your breath.

Stay sitting upright and slowly rotate your head to look straight ahead.

It is important to hold the position for at least 30 seconds or until nystagmus stops before moving to step seven.

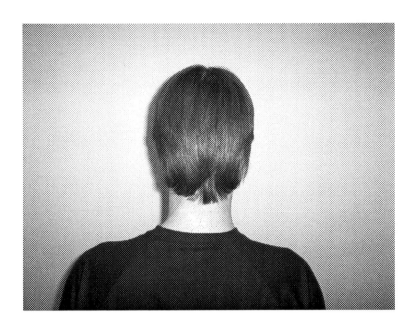

17-1 "Step Seven"

*Most importantly, the patient MUST stay upright and NOT recline below a 45 degree angle for 48 hours after performing the sequential exercises.

This allows the otoconia to settle and become reabsorbed or reattached to their correct position in the utricle of the inner ear.

It is also advised to use two pillows when you sleep, avoid sleeping on your side and limit end range of motion for cervical extension and flexion for at least one week.

The steps may be repeated if vertigo becomes worse as this is a sign that there are still some free-floating otoconia.

Chapter 18

TEMPORAL MANDIBULAR JOINT
DYSFUNCTION–PROVEN TECHNIQUES

I. **Preparations:**
   A. ALL of the contraindications, precautions, indications, goals/and effects listed in Chapter 2 apply to the proven exercise techniques in this chapter.

II. **Temporal Mandibular Joint Dysfunction Background:**
   34,63,64,70,107,123
   A. The Temporal Mandibular Joint (TMJ) is the ONLY bilateral joint in the body.
      1. The TMJ articulates and moves bilaterally with all motions of opening, closing, translation forward, backward, and side to side.
   B. An often overlooked cause of headaches is often due to TMJ dysfunction.
   C. Many malocclusions of the jaw and teeth also cause TMJ dysfunction.
   D. The anatomy of the TMJ includes a unique fibrous meniscus that translates between the Mandible and the Temporalis interface.
      1. Many times this fibrous meniscus becomes inflamed and/or stretched causing a "popping" sound on opening or closing the mouth.
   E. Pain and localized swelling of the TMJ joint(s) respond favorably to ultrasound, electrical stimulation and cryotherapy modalities in addition to 6 proven therapeutic exercises.

III. **Proven Temporal Mandibular Joint Therapeutic Exercises:** 34,63,64,70,107,123
   A. Mariano Rocobado researched and developed a system of proven exercises for successful TMJ dysfunction rehabilitation.

B. These exercises are known as the "6 × 6" exercises performed 6 repetitions and 6 times a day as follows:

18-1 "Tongue Rest Position & Nasal Breathing"

Make a "clucking" sound with your tongue.
Gently hold ⅓ of the end of your tongue in the position against the roof
   of your mouth at the place it rests to make the "cluck".
Breathe in through your nose and stick out your stomach.
Then breathe out through your nose and pull in your stomach.

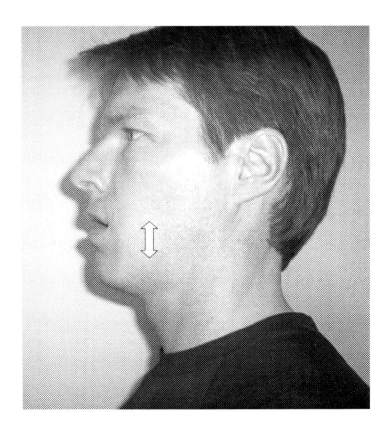

Perform 6 repetitions 6 times a day as tolerated.

18-2 "Controlled Opening"

Place your tongue in the same position as described in 18-1.
Open your mouth only as far as you can without your tongue leaving
the roof of your mouth.

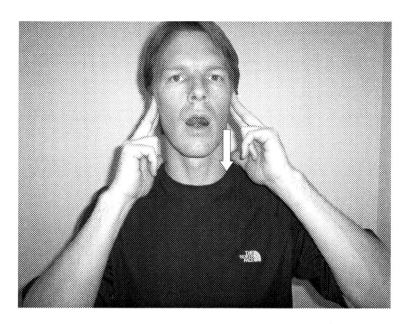

Perform 6 repetitions 6 times a day as tolerated.

*The amount of jaw opening is also recommended for chewing
functions.

18-3 "Rhythmic Stabilization"

Place the tongue in the rest position described in exercise 18-1.
Grasp your chin with one hand.
Apply resistance sideways to the right and then to the left.
Apply resistance toward opening and then toward closing the mouth.
Maintain the same jaw position at all times.

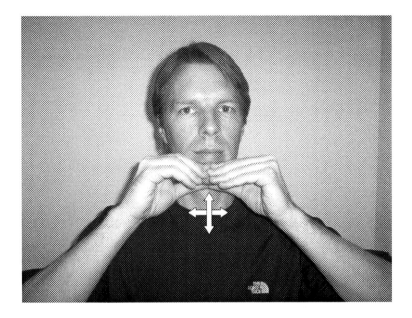

Perform the side/side and open/close isometric exercises 6 repetitions
   6 times a day as tolerated.

18-4 "Stabilized Head Flexion"

Place both hands with interlocked fingers behind your neck.
Keep your head upright.
Nod your head forward keeping the mouth closed.

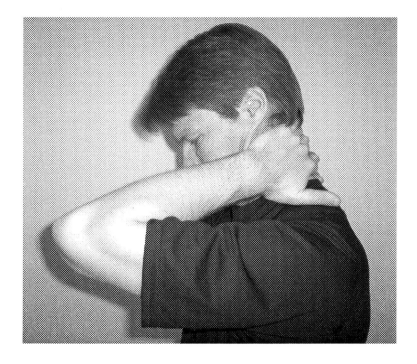

Perform 6 repetitions 6 times a day as tolerated.

18-5 "Chin Tucks"

Do not hold your breath.
Push your chin straight back/elongate the neck
Keep your eyes focused straight ahead.

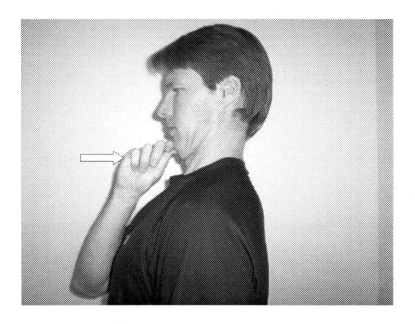

Perform 6 repetitions 6 times a day as tolerated.

18-6 "Shoulder Squeeze"

Do not hold your breath.
Press/retract your shoulder blades together

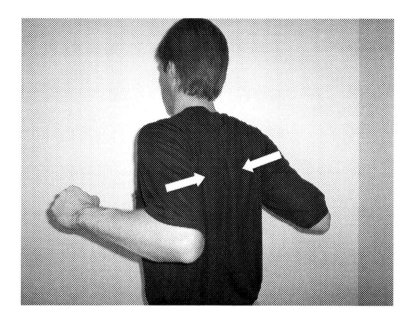

Perform 6 repetitions 6 times a day as tolerated.

Chapter 19

OSTEOPOROSIS – PROVEN
TECHNIQUES

I. **Preparations:**
   A. ALL of the contraindications, precautions, indications, goals/and effects listed in Chapter 2 apply to the proven exercise techniques in this chapter.

II. **Osteoporosis Background:**[34,47,63,64,60,123]
   A. Osteoporosis affects the largest cohort of postmenopausal women between the ages of 50 and 65 years.
   B. Compression fractures in the spine and hip in combination with a forward head posture with thoracic kyphosis or "Dowager's Hump" are telltale signs of advanced osteoporosis.
   C. Bone density testing is commonly used to diagnose osteoporosis.
   D. Hormones, calcium and other medications are often administered to reduce the effects of osteoporosis.
   E. However, therapeutic exercise is the number one treatment for reversing the effects of osteoporosis.
   F. The key to ALL proven Osteoporosis exercises with the exception of postural exercises is weight bearing which is also referred to as, "Bone Loading."

III. **Proven Osteoporosis Therapeutic Exercises:**[34,47,63,64,60,123]
   A. While there are hundreds of researchers who have tested the efficacy of various exercises on Osteoporosis, no cohort retains exclusive acknowledgement for the following eclectic recommendations known as the "5 × 25" exercises:

19-1 "Chin Tuck Exercises"

Do not hold your breath.
Push your chin straight back/elongate the neck
Keep your eyes focused straight ahead.

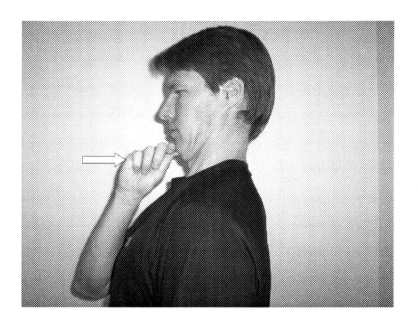

Hold >10 seconds as tolerated.
Relax and repeat 25 times as tolerated.

19-2 **"Shoulder Squeeze"**

Do not hold your breath.
Press/retract your shoulder blades together

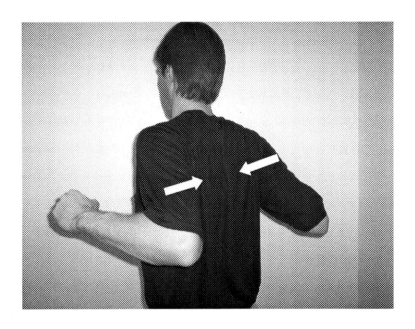

Hold >10 seconds as tolerated.
Relax and repeat 25 times as tolerated.

19-3 **"Prone Press Ups"**

Do not hold your breath.
Relax the back muscles and just use your arms.
Push your body up with your arms, leaving your pelvis flat on the floor.

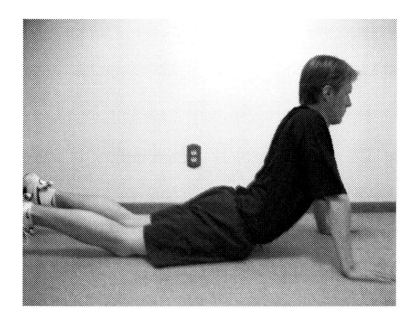

Hold 2 to 5 seconds.
Relax and repeat up to 25 times as tolerated.

19-4 "Mini Wall Slides"

Do NOT hold your breath.
Lean up against a wall.
Slide down the wall about 2 to 4 inches.

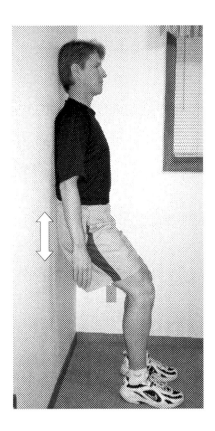

Hold for 2 to 5 seconds.
Then raise up and repeat up to 25 times as tolerated.

*NEVER squat down below a 75 degree bend at the knee.

19-5 "Standing Heel Raises"

Do NOT hold your breath.
Keep your knees extended and raise up on your toes.
Use arm support for maintaining balance as necessary.

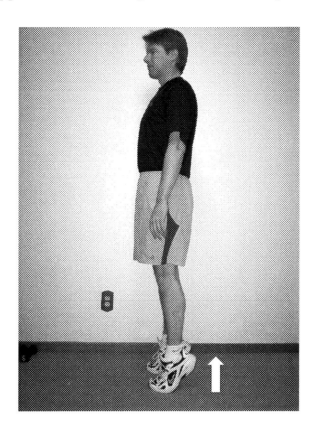

Hold for 2 to 5 seconds.
Then relax and repeat up to 25 times as tolerated.

Chapter 20

PREGNANCY–PROVEN TECHNIQUES

I. **Preparations:** [7,34,47,63,64,70,123,127,136]
    A. ALL of the contraindications, precautions, indications, goals/and effects listed in Chapter 2 apply to the proven exercise techniques in this chapter.
    B. In addition, exercise is contraindicated if any of the following conditions apply:
        1. Incompetent cervix and early dilation.
        2. Substantial vaginal bleeding.
        3. Placenta Previa.
        4. Rupture of membranes and subsequent loss of amniotic fluid.
        5. Premature labor.
        6. Maternal heart disease.
        7. Maternal diabetes or hypertension.
    C. Furthermore, it is important to note that pregnant women should NOT exceed a heart rate of 140 beats per minute while exercising.
    D. Exercise on the back should NOT be performed after the first trimester.
    E. Nearly ALL modalities are strictly contraindicated in pregnant women. Therefore, therapeutic exercise is the choice of treatment in conditions of spinal and lower extremity pain associated with pregnancy.
II. **Pregnancy Background:** [7,34,47,63,64,70,123,127,136]
    A. Approximately 50 percent of ALL pregnant women experience spinal pain.
    B. Nearly 20 percent of these women experience pain so severe that it limits activities of daily living.
    C. The percentage of pregnant women who experience hip, knee and ankle/foot pain also comprise nearly 40 percent.

D. Reasons for the pain associated with pregnancy include:
    1. Increased weight on spinal and lower extremity joints.
    2. Increased joint and ligament laxity due to increased levels of the hormone Relaxin.
    3. Diastasis Recti, the separation of the Rectus Abdominis muscles in the midline at the Linea Alba prevent the abdominal musculature to adequately control the pelvis and lumbar spine.
    4. As the central mass increases, the hips and feet will externally rotate causing a shortening of the Piriformis muscle which often entraps or impinges on the Sciatic nerve causing localized and radiating pain down one or both lower extremities.

III. **Proven Pregnancy Therapeutic Exercises:**[7,34,47,63,64,70,123,127,136]

A. Based on what we know to be contraindicated in pregnancy, as well as the causal factors of spinal and lower extremity pain, there are 7 proven pregnancy therapeutic exercises that are applicable in ALL stages of pregnancy:

20-1 "Chin Tuck Exercises"

Do not hold your breath.
Push your chin straight back/elongate the neck
Keep your eyes focused straight ahead.

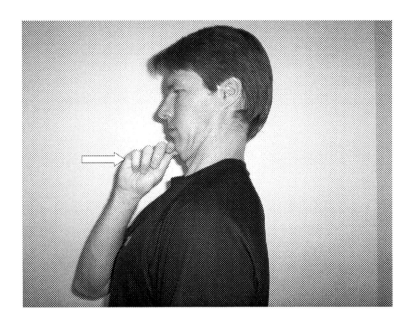

Hold >10 seconds as tolerated.
Relax and repeat 20 to 30 times as tolerated.

20-2 "Rowing"

Do NOT hold your breath.
Start from an extended arm position.
Pull backward using the shoulder blades first, then the arms.

*Do NOT allow your wrists back beyond the vertical plane of the hip

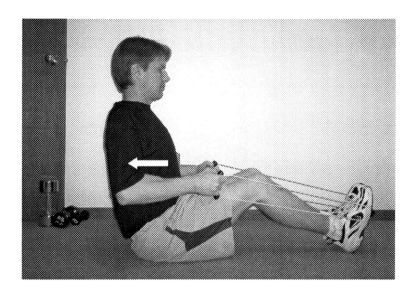

Hold 2 to 5 seconds.
Relax and repeat up to 25 times as tolerated.

20-3 "Posterior Pelvic Tilts"

Do NOT hold your breath.
Rock the pelvis backward and flatten the lumbar spine.
A gentle abdominal crunch contraction often accompanies this
    exercise.

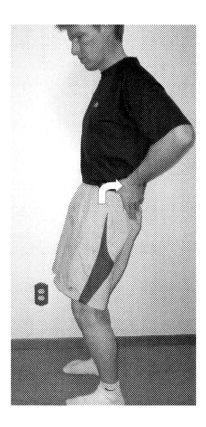

Hold 2 to 5 seconds,
Relax and repeat up to 25 times as tolerated.

20-4 "Mini Wall Slides"

Do NOT hold your breath.
Lean up against a wall.
Slide down the wall about 2 to 4 inches.

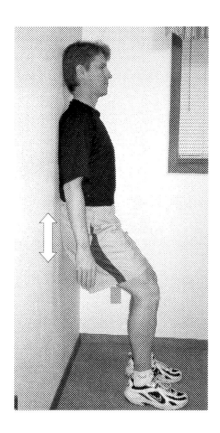

Hold for 2 to 5 seconds.
Then raise up and repeat up to 25 times as tolerated.

*NEVER squat down below a 75 degree bend at the knee.

20-5 "Standing Heel Raises"

Do NOT hold your breath.
Keep your knees extended and raise up on your toes.
Use arm support for maintaining balance as necessary.

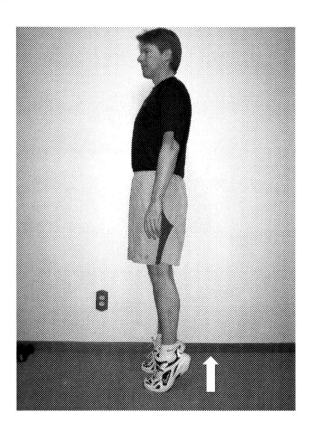

Hold for 2 to 5 seconds.
Then relax and repeat up to 25 times as tolerated.

20-6 "Kegel Exercises"

Kegel's are specially designed to promote bowel and bladder integrity
during the advanced stages of pregnancy.
Instruct the patient to contract the pelvic floor muscles.
This can be practiced and accomplished by starting and stopping uri-
nation flow during elimination activities.

Voluntary contraction of these muscles prevent pregnancy induced incontinence.

They should be performed at least 25 times several times a day and in various positions including standing, sitting and laying.

20-7 "Sitting Piriformis Stretch"

Do NOT hold your breath.
Cross your leg and pull the knee up and across the chest.
Hold 15 to 30 seconds and repeat 3 to 5 times as tolerated.
Repeat on both sides.

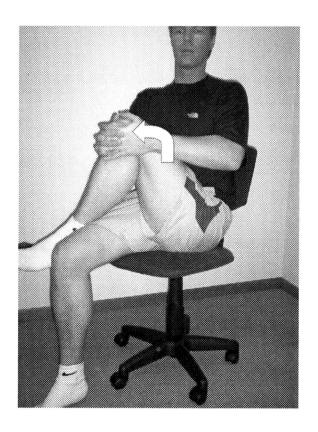

*Note, if central obesity prevents this stretch, you may also cross your leg and push down on the knee to reduce the excess hip and foot external rotation that puts pressure on the sciatic nerve.

Part 6

PROVEN JOINT MOBILIZATION
TECHNIQUES

Chapter 21

PROVEN JOINT
MOBILIZATION TECHNIQUES

I. **General Joint Mobilization Contraindications:**[3,4,34,44,47,51,63,64,70,71,77,100,106,115,123,137]

   A. Common contraindications to joint mobilization includes, but is not limited to:
      1. Increased Inflammation.
      2. Severe Osteoporosis.
      3. Ischemia/Peripheral Vascular Disease (PVD).
      4. Severe Pain Lasting More Than 24 Hours.
      5. Significant Disruption To The Healing Process.
      6. Infection.
      7. Fracture.
      8. Malignancy.
      9. Joint Hypermobility.
      10. Joint Replacement Surgeries.
      11. Positive Vertebral Artery Insufficiency Test (Cervical Spine Mobilizations Only).

II. **General Joint Mobilization Precautions/Red Flags:**[3,4,34,44,47,51,63,64,70,71,77,100,106,115,123,137]

   A. Red Flags for possible visceral pathology (i.e., cancer) include but are not limited to:[25]
      1. Weight Fluctuations.
      2. Inability To Sleep.
      3. Medications Are Required To Sleep.
      4. Pain Becomes Worse With Walking.
      5. Recent Fever Or Infection.

III. **General Joint Mobilization Indications:**[3,4,34,44,47,51,63,64,70,71,77,100,106,115,123,137]

   A. Weakness.
   B. Pain.
   C. Muscle Spasms.

    D.   Musculoskeletal Injury/Trauma.

    E.   Decreased Joint Proprioreception.

    F.   Decreased Range Of Motion.

    G.   Decreased Flexibility.

    H.   Decreased Circulation.

    I.   Impaired Functional (Vocational/Avocational) Activities.

    J.   Swelling/Edema.

IV. **General Joint Mobilization Goals/Benefits:** [3,4,34,44,47,51,63,64,70,71,77,100,106,115,123,137]

    A.   Decreased Pain.

    B.   Decreased Muscle Spasms.

    C.   Increased Range of Motion.

    D.   Increased Flexibility.

    E.   Increased Strength.

    F.   Increased Joint Nutrition.

V. **General Joint Mobilization Considerations:** [34,51,63,64,81,82,94,100,123,124]

    A.   While this is not a book exclusively devoted to joint mobilization, its' importance as an adjunct modality to therapeutic exercise cannot be underestimated.

    B.   Joint Mobilization Convex/Concave Rules:

        1.   Each joint in the body is categorized as one of six types. They are as follows from smallest to largest amounts of movement allowed:

            a.   *Plane* joints allow simple gliding or sliding between two flat surfaces.

                i.   Common examples include the Tibiofibular, Carpometacarpal and Acromioclavicular joints.

            b.   *Hinge* joints allow movement around one axis, usually flexion and extension only.

                i.   Common examples include the Tibiofemoral (Knee) and Interphalangeal joints.

            c.   *Pivot* joints allow movement around one axis pivoting within a bony ring.

                i.   Common examples include the superior and inferior Radioulnar joints.

            d.   *Ellipsoidal* joints allow movement in two directions at right angles to each other. These allow flexion, extension, abduction and adduction but no rotation.

    i.   Common examples include the Radiocarpal
         and Metacarpophalangeal joints.
e.   *Saddle* joints allow movement in two directions at
     right angles to each other. These allow flexion, ex-
     tension, abduction, adduction and the combination
     movement of slight rotation.
    i.   An example of this type of joint is the Carpo-
         metacarpal joint of the thumb.
f.   *Ball and socket* joints allow multiaxial movement in-
     cluding flexion, extension, abduction, adduction,
     medial rotation, lateral rotation and circumduction.
    i.   Common examples of this type of joint are the
         Glenohumeral (Shoulder) and Iliofemoral (Hip)
         joints.
2.   For each joint and associated movement there is one
     facet that is convex (bowed out) and one facet that is
     concave (bowed in).
3.   The rules that govern the direction of joint mobilization
     forces are based on the physical structure of the joint
     and desired direction of increased range of motion.
4.   Effective joint mobilizations essentially consist of "Glid-
     ing" which is a combination of two movements:
a.   *Sliding* which is characterized by one bone sliding
     perpendicular to the other.
    i.   In a situation where the joint being moved is
         concave and the stabilized joint is convex, slid-
         ing occurs in the SAME direction as the desired
         increase in range of motion.
    ii. For example, when the Metacarpal Phalangeal
         joint requires more extension, the Metacarpal
         is convex and stabilized while the Proximal
         Phalange concave slide direction is moved
         dorsally/posteriorly.
    iii. In a situation where the joint being moved is
         convex and the stabilized joint is concave, slid-
         ing occurs in the OPPOSITE direction as the
         desired increase in range of motion.
    iv. For example, when the Glenohumeral joint re-
         quires more flexion, the Scapula which is con-

cave is stabilized while the Humerus convex slide direction is directed inferiorly.

b. *Rolling* which is characterized by one bone rolling on another. Essentially this is how the majority of joint range of motion occurs.

    i.   Rolling joint mobilization forces always occur in the SAME direction as the desired increase in range of motion.

c. *Gliding* is the combination of two mobilization forces acting on a joint simultaneously, or nearly simultaneously.

    i.   In the situation where the concave joint is being moved on a stabilized convex joint, the gliding forces are in the SAME direction as the desired increase in range of motion.

    ii. For example, the slide component and roll component of joint mobilization force are both directed dorsally/posteriorly in the Metacarpal Phalangeal joint to increase extension.

    iii. In the situation where the convex joint is being moved on a stabilized concave joint, the gliding forces are in the OPPOSITE direction as the desired increase in range of motion.

    iv. For example, the slide component of joint mobilization force is directed inferiorly while the roll component is directed superiorly in the Glenohumeral joint to increase flexion.

C. Joint Mobilization Grading Scale:

1. GRADE 1:

    a.   Small amplitude, rhythmic oscillation at the beginning of joint range of motion.. Also known as "Joint Support."

2. GRADE 2:

    a.   Large amplitude, rhythmic oscillation within the joint range of motion, but not reaching the limit.

3. GRADE 3:

    a.   Large amplitude, rhythmic oscillation up to the limit of available joint range of motion and stressed into tissue resistance.

4. GRADE 4:
   a. Small amplitude, rhythmic oscillation at the limit of joint range of motion and stressed into tissue resistance.
5. GRADE 5:
   a. Small amplitude, high velocity thrust to break adhesions reserved for the end limit of available motion.

D. Joint Mobilization Efficacy Rules:
   1. Position the patient for comfort and appropriately drape the patient.
   2. Explain the procedure to the patient.
   3. Assess the area to be mobilized for any contra-indications.
   4. Do NOT perform more than 15 to 20 grade 3+ mobilizations to the same joint in the same direction without allowing at least 48 hours of rest between treatments.
   5. Document the patient's tolerance to treatment, area/joint(s) treated, grade of mobilization, and number of mobilization oscillations in a particular area.
   6. The treating clinician should use good body mechanics and position themselves where they do NOT have to reach or hunch their shoulders.
   7. ALWAYS block the joints above and below the level you are mobilizing in order to isolate the mobilization forces to the joint being treated.
   8. Joint mobilizations should be performed prior to stretching.
   9. Slight joint distraction increases the comfort level of joint mobilizations while performing the glide movements.
   10. Joint mobilizations MUST be performed in the "Loose Packed Position" where the joint is not bound by muscular, ligament or other tissue.
   11. Although joint mobilizations are generally contraindicated for patients with joint replacement surgeries, some physicians allow grade 2 to 3 mobilizations when capsular tightness limits passive range of motion.
   12. Warm and clean hands are always a big hit with your patients.

Chapter 22

PROVEN JOINT MOBILIZATION
TECHNIQUES–UPPER EXTREMITY

I. **Upper Extremity Joint Mobilization Preparations:**
   A. Following all of the joint mobilization considerations in
      Chapter 21, we will now look at the most efficacious joint
      mobilizations for the most common upper extremity
      diagnoses/problems.

II. **Shoulder Mobilizations:**[34,51,63,64,81,94,123,124]
   A. Most common problems with joint capsular range of mo-
      tion limitations in the Glenohumeral joint involve decreased
      flexion, abduction and external rotation.
   B. The shoulder should be positioned in the loose packed posi-
      tion which is defined as 55 degrees of shoulder abduction
      and 30 degrees of horizontal adduction (i.e., Plane of the
      Scapula).
   C. The convex Humerus will be moved on the stabilized con-
      cave Glenoid Fossa/Scapula.

20-8 "Shoulder Flexion Mobilization"

Do not allow the patient to hold their breath.
Apply slight distraction force.
Direct the slide component inferiorly and the roll component
   superiorly.
Oscillate at the end of tolerable range of motion as delineated by
   the grading scale.
Relax and repeat as tolerated.

20-9 "Shoulder Abduction Mobilization"

Do not allow the patient to hold their breath.

Apply slight distraction force.

Direct the slide component inferiorly and laterally while the roll component superiorly.

Oscillate at the end of tolerable range of motion as delineated by the grading scale.

Relax and repeat as tolerated.

20-10 "Shoulder External Rotation Mobilization"

Do not allow the patient to hold their breath.

Apply slight distraction force.

Direct the slide component anteriorly and the roll component posteriorly/externally.

Oscillate at the end of tolerable range of motion as delineated by the grading scale.

Relax and repeat as tolerated.

III. **Elbow and Forearm Mobilizations:**[34,51,63,64,81,94,123,124]
   A. Most common problems with joint capsular range of motion limitations in the Humeroulnar and Humeroradial joints involve decreased elbow extension whereas the Radioulnar joints involve decreased Supination and Pronation.
   B. The elbow should be positioned in the loose packed position which is defined as 70 degrees of flexion and 10 degrees of Supination.
   C. The concave Radius/Ulna will be moved on the stabilized convex Humerus for increasing elbow extension.

20-11 "Elbow Extension Mobilization"

Do not allow the patient to hold their breath.

Apply slight distraction force.

Direct the slide and roll components inferiorly/posteriorly.

Oscillate at the end of tolerable range of motion as delineated by the grading scale.

Relax and repeat as tolerated.

     D.   The convex Radius will be moved on the stabilized concave Ulna in the Proximal Radioulnar joint for increasing forearm Supination.

20-12 "Forearm Supination Mobilization"

Do not allow the patient to hold their breath.

Apply slight distraction force.

Direct the slide component medially/anteriorly and roll component laterally/posteriorly on the Radius.

Oscillate at the end of tolerable range of motion as delineated by the grading scale.

Relax and repeat as tolerated.

20-13 "Forearm Pronation Mobilization"

Do not allow the patient to hold their breath.

Apply slight distraction force.

Direct the slide component laterally/posteriorly and roll component medially/anteriorly on the Radius.

Oscillate at the end of tolerable range of motion as delineated by the grading scale.

Relax and repeat as tolerated.

IV. **Wrist, Hand and Finger Mobilizations:**[34,51,63,64,81,94,123,124]
     A.   Most common problems with joint capsular range of motion limitations in the Radiocarpal, Metacarpophalageal, and Interphalangeal joints involve decreased flexion and extension.
     B.   The wrist and fingers should be positioned in the loose packed position which is defined as 15 degrees of wrist extension and 10 degrees of Metacarpophalangeal and Interphalangeal flexion.
     C.   The convex Carpals will be moved on the stabilized concave Distal Radioulnar joint in the wrist.

20-14 "Wrist Flexion Mobilization"

Do not allow the patient to hold their breath.

Apply slight distraction force.

Direct the slide component superiorly/dorsally and the roll component inferiorly/ventrally.

Oscillate at the end of tolerable range of motion as delineated by the grading scale.

Relax and repeat as tolerated.

20-15 "Wrist Extension Mobilization"

Do not allow the patient to hold their breath.

Apply slight distraction force.

Direct the slide component inferiorly/ventrally and the roll component superiorly/dorsally.

Oscillate at the end of tolerable range of motion as delineated by the grading scale.

Relax and repeat as tolerated.

      D.   The concave Proximal Interphalangeal joint will be moved on the stabilized convex Metacarpals in the hand.

20-16 "Metacarpophalangeal Flexion Mobilization"

Do not allow the patient to hold their breath.

Apply slight distraction force.

Direct the slide and roll components inferiorly/ventrally.

Oscillate at the end of tolerable range of motion as delineated by the grading scale.

Relax and repeat as tolerated.

20-17 "Metacarpophalangeal Extension Mobilization"

Do not allow the patient to hold their breath.

Apply slight distraction force.

Direct the slide and roll components superiorly/dorsally.

Oscillate at the end of tolerable range of motion as delineated by the grading scale.

Relax and repeat as tolerated.

      E.   The concave Middle or Distal Phalanges will be moved on the stabilized convex Proximal or Middle Phalanges.

20-18 "Phalangeal Flexion Mobilization"

Do not allow the patient to hold their breath.
Apply slight distraction force.
Direct the slide and roll components inferiorly/ventrally.
Oscillate at the end of tolerable range of motion as delineated by the
grading scale.
Relax and repeat as tolerated.

20-19 "Phalangeal Extension Mobilization"

Do not allow the patient to hold their breath.
Apply slight distraction force.
Direct the slide and roll components superiorly/dorsally.
Oscillate at the end of tolerable range of motion as delineated by the
grading scale.
Relax and repeat as tolerated.

Chapter 23

PROVEN JOINT MOBILIZATION TECHNIQUES – LOWER EXTREMITY

I. **Lower Extremity Joint Mobilization Preparations:**
   A. Following all of the joint mobilization considerations in Chapter 21, we will now look at the most efficacious joint mobilizations for the most common lower extremity diagnoses/problems.

II. **Hip Mobilizations:**[34,51,63,64,81,94,123,124]
   A. Most common problems with joint capsular range of motion limitations in the Iliofemoral joint involve decreased flexion and extension.
   B. The hip should be positioned in the loose packed position which is defined as 30 degrees of hip flexion, 30 degrees of abduction and slight external rotation.
   C. The convex Femur will be moved on the stabilized concave Acetabulum of the Ilia.

23-1 "Hip Flexion Mobilization"

Do not allow the patient to hold their breath.

Apply slight distraction force.

Direct the slide component posteriorly and the roll component anteriorly.

Oscillate at the end of tolerable range of motion as delineated by the grading scale.

Relax and repeat as tolerated.

23-2 "Hip Extension Mobilization"

Do not allow the patient to hold their breath.

Apply slight distraction force.

Direct the slide component anteriorly and the roll component
   posteriorly.
Oscillate at the end of tolerable range of motion as delineated by
   the grading scale.
Relax and repeat as tolerated.

III. **Knee Mobilizations:**[34,51,63,64,81,94,123,124]
   A.   Most common problems with joint capsular range of motion
         limitations in the Tibiofemoral joint involve decreased knee
         flexion and extension.
   B.   The knee should be positioned in the loose packed position
         which is defined as 25 degrees of flexion.
   C.   The concave Tibia will be moved on the stabilized convex
         Femur for increasing knee flexion and extension.

23-3 "Knee Flexion Mobilization"

Do not allow the patient to hold their breath.
Apply slight distraction force.
Direct the slide and roll components posteriorly.
Oscillate at the end of tolerable range of motion as delineated by the
   grading scale.
Relax and repeat as tolerated.

23-4 "Knee Extension Mobilization"

Do not allow the patient to hold their breath.
Apply slight distraction force.
Direct the slide and roll components anteriorly.
Oscillate at the end of tolerable range of motion as delineated by the
   grading scale.
Relax and repeat as tolerated.

IV. **Ankle, Foot and Toe Mobilizations:**[34,51,63,64,81,94,123,124]
   A.   Most common problems with joint capsular range of motion
         limitations in the Talocrural joint include decreased plan-
         tarflexion, dorsiflexion and eversion. In addition, decreased
         flexion and extension of the Metatarsalphalangeal joints
         commonly occur.

B. The ankle should be positioned in the loose packed position which is defined as 10 degrees of plantarflexion.

C. In the Talocrural (ankle) joint, the convex Talus will be moved on the stabilized concave Mortice which is made up of the Tibia and Fibula.

23-5 "Ankle Dorsiflexion Mobilization"

Do not allow the patient to hold their breath.

Apply slight distraction force.

Direct the slide component frontally/anteriorly and the roll component superiorly.

Oscillate at the end of tolerable range of motion as delineated by the grading scale.

Relax and repeat as tolerated.

23-6 "Ankle Plantarflexion Mobilization"

Do not allow the patient to hold their breath.

Apply slight distraction force.

Direct the slide component inferiorly/ventrally and the roll component superiorly/dorsally.

Oscillate at the end of tolerable range of motion as delineated by the grading scale.

Relax and repeat as tolerated.

23-7 "Ankle Eversion Mobilization"

Do not allow the patient to hold their breath.

Apply slight distraction force.

Direct the slide component medially and the roll component laterally.

Oscillate at the end of tolerable range of motion as delineated by the grading scale.

Relax and repeat as tolerated.

D. In the Metatarsalphalangeal joints, the concave Proximal Interphalangeal joint will be moved on the stabilized convex Metatarsals of the foot.

23-8 "Metatarsalphalangeal Flexion Mobilization"

Do not allow the patient to hold their breath.
Apply slight distraction force.
Direct the slide and roll components inferiorly/ventrally.
Oscillate at the end of tolerable range of motion as delineated by the
   grading scale.
Relax and repeat as tolerated.

23-9 "Metatarsalphalangeal Extension Mobilization"

Do not allow the patient to hold their breath.
Apply slight distraction force.
Direct the slide and roll components superiorly/dorsally.
Oscillate at the end of tolerable range of motion as delineated by the
   grading scale.
Relax and repeat as tolerated.

Chapter 24

PROVEN JOINT MOBILIZATION
TECHNIQUES – SPINE

I. **Spinal Joint Mobilization General Considerations:**[34,51,63,64,81,94,100,112,123,124]

    A. The same joint mobilization contraindications, precautions, indications, goals/effects listed in Chapter 21 apply to the spine.

    B. However, the complex biomechanics of the spine predicate a different approach to proven mobilization techniques in this body region.

    C. The spine and pelvis have over 60 bones and 100 joint articulations.

    D. Fryette's Laws of Spinal Motion' make up the basis for joint mobility of individual vertebral segments.

        1. *Law I:* For the thoracic and lumbar spine, in neutral spinal mechanics, side-bending and rotation are to OPPOSITE sides for a vertebral segment.

        2. *Law II:* In all conditions for the cervical spine (C3-7) as well as in non-neutral mechanics for the thoracic and lumbar spine, side-bending and rotation are to the SAME sides for a vertebral segment.

        3. *Law III:* Motion introduced in one plane at any vertebral segment reduces available motions in other planes at that segment.

    E. The challenge of applying Fryette's laws of spinal motion in clinical settings make it difficult for clinician's to accurately ascertain the motion of individual spinal segments. Therefore, we have collected the "Proven Joint Mobilization" techniques from research literature in order to simplify the process.

311

II. **Spinal Joint Mobilization Preparations:** [34,51,63,64,81,94,100,112,123,124]

   A. Following all of the joint mobilization considerations in Chapter 21, we will now look at the most efficacious joint mobilizations for the most common spinal diagnoses/problems.

   B. It is ESSENTIAL that a Vertebral Artery Test is performed and found to be negative prior to performing ANY joint mobilization techniques in the cervical spine.

   C. The technique of *Muscle Energy* is also widely utilized and proven effective in spinal mobilization techniques. These techniques may also be utilized in the extremity mobilizations, however research data regarding its' efficacy is scant and therefore beyond the scope of this text.

   1. The Muscle Energy technique involves the reversal of a muscle's origin and insertion.

   2. Essentially Muscle Energy is a gentle isometric contraction in the same or opposite direction(s) of end range of motion.

   a. For example, to increase cervical rotation to the left, the clinician will rotate the patient's head to the end range of motion of left cervical rotation. At that point the clinician will provide isometric resistance and instruct the patient to contract, or try and rotate the head left or right depending on the purpose and position of the spinal segment.

   b. Other proven Muscle Energy examples will be cited in the applicable techniques sections below.

III. **Cervical Spine Mobilizations:** [34,51,63,64,81,94,100,112,123,124]

   A. Most common problems with joint capsular range of motion limitations in the cervical spine are easily assessed with the patient lying supine and performing gentle lateral gliding side to side for each cervical segment.

   1. To isolate individual cervical segments, it is advisable to begin in an extended position for C3 and incrementally increase the amount of cervical flexion to lock down and isolate the individual segments of C4-C7 according to Fryette's Laws of spinal motion. Proficiency in these isolation techniques is accomplished with considerable practice.

2. Once a segment of segment(s) are found to be re-
    stricted, the gross range of motion limitations in
    sidebending will correspond with limitations in lateral
    cervical segmental mobility.

24-1 "Cervical Left Sidebending/Right Lateral Mobilization C3-4"

Do not allow the patient to hold their breath.
Apply slight distraction force.
Passively move the cervical spine to the end range of motion for left
    sidebending.
(Provide incremental cervical flexion to isolate lower segments from
    C3-7)
Direct the segmental glide components laterally to the right on the lim-
    ited segment with counterforce on the cranium to the left.
Oscillate at the end of tolerable range of motion as delineated by the
    grading scale.
Relax and repeat as tolerated.

24-2 "Cervical Right Sidebending/Left Lateral Mobilization C7-8"

Do not allow the patient to hold their breath.
Apply slight distraction force.
Passively move the cervical spine to the end range of motion for right
    sidebending.
(Provide incremental cervical flexion to isolate lower segments from
    C3-7)
Direct the segmental glide components laterally to the left on the lim-
    ited segment with counterforce on the cranium to the right.
Oscillate at the end of tolerable range of motion as delineated by the
    grading scale.
Relax and repeat as tolerated.

B. For limitations in cervical rotation, one should look primar-
    ily to the C2 joint which provides over 50 percent of cervical
    rotation range of motion.

C. The patient should be supine and the cervical spine extended. Muscle energy techniques are applied in this position and may be directed isometrically in either direction right or left depending on patient tolerance.

24-3 "Cervical Left Rotation Muscle Energy C2"

Do not allow the patient to hold their breath.

Apply slight distraction force.

Passively move the cervical spine to the end range of motion for left rotation.

(Keep the cervical spine in an extended position)

Isometrically hold the cranium and direct the patient to isometrically contract or push against a right or left rotational force depending on patient tolerance.

Relax and repeat as tolerated.

24-4 "Cervical Right Rotation Muscle Energy C2"

Do not allow the patient to hold their breath.

Apply slight distraction force.

Passively move the cervical spine to the end range of motion for right rotation.

(Keep the cervical spine in an extended position)

Isometrically hold the cranium and direct the patient to isometrically contract or push against a right or left rotational force depending on patient tolerance.

Relax and repeat as tolerated.

IV. **Thoracic Spine Mobilizations:**[34,51,63,64,81,94,100,112,123,124]
   A. Most common problems with facet joint capsular range of motion limitations in the thoracic spine are easily assessed with the patient lying prone and performing gentle posterior/anterior gliding side to side for each thoracic segment.
      1. Limitations in anterior movement and/or complaints of pain and muscle guarding are tell tale signs of hypomobility in the thoracic spine.
      2. Three proven thoracic spine mobilization techniques are detailed below and are rank ordered from most segmentally specific to least segmentally specific.

24-5 "Thoracic Anterior Mobilization Prone"

This is the most segmentally specific thoracic mobilization technique.
Do not allow the patient to hold their breath.
Apply unilateral or bilateral anterior directional force on the specific thoracic facet joint that is hypomobile.
Oscillate at the end of tolerable range of motion as delineated by the grading scale.
Relax and repeat as tolerated.

24-6 "Thoracic Anterior Mobilization Supine"

Although less segmentally specific, it is generally more tolerable for female patients that the prone technique.
Do not allow the patient to hold their breath.
Have the patient cross their arms and actively grab their shoulders.
Place your fist palm up (Thenar eminence and Proximal Interphalangeal Joints provide bilateral anterior mobilization force) over the thoracic facet joints (usually 3 or 4 segments are mobilized with this technique at a time) that are hypomobile.
Have the patient lay supine on your fist on a flat surface and direct mobilization forces superiorly/posteriorly through the elbows of the patient.
Oscillate at the end of tolerable range of motion as delineated by the grading scale.
Relax and repeat as tolerated.

24-7 "Thoracic Distraction Mobilization Sitting/Standing"

Although less segmentally specific, it is appropriate for patients who cannot tolerate mobilization techniques in the prone or supine positions.
Do not allow the patient to hold their breath.
Have the patient cross their arms and actively grab their shoulders.
With the patient sitting or standing, grab around the patient from behind and focus superior distraction force through the elbows of the patient.
(To include an increased anterior mobilization force you may use a rolled up towel between the clinician's chest and the patient's back)
Oscillate at the end of tolerable range of motion as delineated by the grading scale.
Relax and repeat as tolerated.

V. **Lumbar Spine Mobilizations:**[34,51,63,64,81,94,100,112,123,124]
    A. Most common problems with facet joint capsular range of
        motion limitations in the lumbar spine are easily assessed
        through range of motion limitations when comparing right
        to left or anterior to posterior planes.
        1. Due to the biomechanics of the lumbar spine, the mo-
            tion of rotation involves combination movements of
            flexion/extension and lateral sidebending.
        2. The proven lumbar spine mobilization techniques are
            detailed below can involve muscle energy techniques
            ALWAYS applied in the OPPOSITE direction of the
            mobilization/range of motion force.
        3. The amount of lumbar flexion or extension in these
            proven lumbar spine mobilization techniques is depen-
            dent on isolating a specific segment of the lumbar spine
            (L1-5) and/or treating specific flexion/extension range
            of motion limitations in the lumbar spine.

24-8 "Lumbar Right Rotation Mobilization"

Do not allow the patient to hold their breath.
Have the patient lay on their left side with their knee flexed up and
    across their body.
Then instruct the patient to reach back with their right arm and at-
    tempt to lay it on the plinth.
Position the patient in the desired amount of lumbar flexion or
    extension.
The counterforce positions of the clinician's hands are applied on the
    right shoulder (left hand) and the right ilium (right hand).
Oscillate at the end of tolerable range of motion as delineated by the
    grading scale.
(You may also use Muscle Energy techniques by holding the counter-
    force positions and instructing the patient to isometrically contract
    and try to push their right hip to the floor)
Relax and repeat as tolerated.

24-9 "Lumbar Left Rotation Mobilization"

Do not allow the patient to hold their breath.

Have the patient lay on their right side with their knee flexed up and across their body.

Then instruct the patient to reach back with their left arm and attempt to lay it on the plinth/floor.

Position the patient in the desired amount of lumbar flexion or extension.

The counterforce positions of the clinician's hands are applied on the left shoulder (right hand) and the left ilium (left hand).

Oscillate at the end of tolerable range of motion as delineated by the grading scale.

(You may also use Muscle Energy techniques by holding the counter-force positions and instructing the patient to isometrically contract and try to push their left hip to the floor)

Relax and repeat as tolerated.

VI. **Sacral-Iliac Spine Mobilizations:**[34,51,63,64,81,94,100,112,123,124]
  A. Most common problems with facet joint capsular range of motion limitations in the sacral-iliac (pelvis) spine are difficult to assess due to the very small movements involved.
  B. However, tell tale signs of sacral-iliac spinal range of motion limitations involve a traumatic mechanism of injury such as falling to the ground or stepping off a curb wrong, and show up in evaluation as an antalgic gait and/or localized point tenderness and swelling.
    1. Applying empirically derived research here, I have seen the majority of sacral-iliac dysfunctions in patients between the ages of 30 and 60 years.
    2. This is primarily due to the fact that the pelvis fuses in nearly all patients over the age of 60 years, whereas patients below 30 years of age have enough mobility to self-correct.
    3. The application of proven sacral-iliac joint mobilization techniques is a four step process outlined below. Specific diagnoses may predicate the continued individual use of certain mobilization procedures in addition to the sequential methodology.

4. Muscle Energy techniques are ALWAYS utilized in sacral-iliac joint mobilizations and the direction of Muscle Energy force is ALWAYS applied in the OPPO-SITE direction of the mobilization/range of motion force.

24-10 "Sacral-Iliac Distraction Mobilization"

This is ALWAYS performed first in the Sacral-Iliac mobilization sequence.
Do not allow the patient to hold their breath.
Have the patient lay on their back with their knee flexed up and feet flat on the floor or plinth.
Position your fists side by side between the patient's knees.
Then instruct the patient to push as hard as they can against your fists and hold 5 seconds.
Repeat the contract-relax Muscle Energy technique 5 times.

24-11 "Sacral-Iliac Flexion Mobilization"

This is performed in the case of limited pelvic flexion and may be performed unilaterally in the case of one-sided dysfunction, or bilaterally in the case of general sacral-iliac flexion hypomobility.
Do not allow the patient to hold their breath.
Have the patient lay on their back and keep one knee flexed with the foot on the floor or plinth. Allow the leg on the treated side to fall flat or dangle off the edge of the plinth.
In this extended leg position instruct the patient to lift their knee up against your hand and hold the isometric contraction 5 seconds.
Repeat the contract-relax Muscle Energy technique 5 times.
(Perform this technique on the other side as indicated)

24-12 "Sacral-Iliac Extension Mobilization"

This is performed in the case of limited pelvic extension and may be performed unilaterally in the case of one-sided dysfunction, or bilaterally in the case of general sacral-iliac flexion hypomobility.
Do not allow the patient to hold their breath.

Have the patient lay on their back and start with their hip and knee
   flexed in a 90/90 position. Allow the untreated leg to fall flat or
   dangle off the edge of the plinth.
In this flexed leg position instruct the patient to push against your
   shoulder and hold the isometric contraction 5 seconds.
Repeat the contract-relax Muscle Energy technique 5 times.
(Perform this technique on the other side as indicated)

24-13 "Sacral-Iliac Approximation Mobilization"

This is ALWAYS performed last in the Sacral-Iliac mobilization
   sequence.
Do not allow the patient to hold their breath.
Have the patient lay on their back with their knee flexed up and feet
   flat on the floor or plinth.
Position your hands on the outsides of the patient's knees and hold
   them together.
Then instruct the patient to push as hard as they can against your
   hands and hold 5 seconds.
Repeat the contract-relax Muscle Energy technique 5 times.

Part 7

PROVEN MASSAGE TECHNIQUES

Chapter 25

PROVEN MASSAGE TECHNIQUES

I. **General Massage Contraindications:** [3,4,34,44,47,51,63,64,70,71, 77,106,115,123,137]

   A. Common contraindications to massage includes, but is not limited to: [12,14,19,26]
   1. Increased Inflammation.
   2. Severe Osteoporosis.
   3. Ischemia/Peripheral Vascular Disease (PVD).
   4. Severe Pain Lasting More Than 24 Hours.
   5. Positive (+) Homan's Test for Deep Vein Thrombosis.
   6. Significant Disruption To The Healing Process.
   7. Infection.
   8. Fracture.
   9. Hematoma's.
   10. Malignancy.
   11. Skin Diseases.

II. **General Massage Precautions/Red Flags:** [3,4,34,44,47,51,63, 64,70,71,77,106,115,123,137]

   A. Red Flags for possible visceral pathology (i.e., cancer) include but are not limited to: [25]
   1. Weight Fluctuations.
   2. Inability To Sleep.
   3. Medications Are Required To Sleep.
   4. Pain Becomes Worse With Walking.
   5. Recent Fever Or Infection.
   B. Other precautions include:
   1. Delayed Onset Muscle Soreness (DOMS).
   2. Overtraining/Overwork.
   3. Severe Osteoporosis.
   4. Degree of Ischemia/Peripheral Vascular Disease (PVD).
   5. Steroid Use.

     6.   Age.

     7.   Avoiding Valsalva Maneuver.

III. **General Massage Indications:**[3,4,34,44,47,51,63,64,70,71,77,106,115,123,137]

    A.   Weakness.

    B.   Pain.

    C.   Muscle Spasms.

    D.   Musculoskeletal Injury/Trauma.

    E.   Decreased Joint Proprioreception.

    F.   Decreased Range Of Motion.

    G.   Decreased Flexibility.

    H.   Decreased Circulation.

    I.   Impaired Functional (Vocational/Avocational) Activities.

    J.   Swelling/Edema.

IV. **General Massage Goals/Benefits:**[3,4,34,44,47,51,63,64,70,71,77,106,115,123,137]

    A.   Decreased Pain.

    B.   Decreased Muscle Spasms.

    C.   Decreased Swelling.

    D.   Increased Strength.

    E.   Increased Range of Motion.

    F.   Increased Flexibility.

    G.   Increased Circulation.

V. **General Massage Considerations:**[17,23,72,122]

    A.   While this is not a book exclusively devoted to massage, its' importance as an adjunct modality to therapeutic exercise cannot be underestimated.

    B.   Massage Efficacy Rules:

        1.   Position the patient for comfort and appropriately drape the patient.

        2.   NEVER massage over or near the breast/genital areas.

        3.   Explain the procedure to the patient.

        4.   Assess the area to be massaged for any contraindications.

        5.   Perform the treatment NOT to exceed 20 minutes in one area as swelling will become a factor.

        6.   Document the patient's tolerance to treatment, type of massage utilized, and length of treatment time in a particular area.

7. The treating clinician should use good body mechanics and position themselves where they do NOT have to reach or hunch their shoulders.

8. Warm and clean hands are always a big hit with your massage patients.

VI. **Proven Massage Techniques:** [17,23,72,122]

A. There are several types of basic massage techniques within two major categories:

1. "Soft" Massage Techniques are generally classified as Effleurage; Shingles; Fulling; Swedish; and other popular types that primarily decrease pain and muscle spasm.

2. "Hard" Massage Techniques are generally classified as Petrissage; Knuckling; Shiatsu, Myofascial Release, Friction, Tapotement; and other popular types that primarily stretch contracted or spasmodic tissues.

B. *Effleurage* is a "soft" massage technique where you glide over the skin with a lubricating interface medium.

1. The lubricating interface medium should be hypoallergenic.

2. Although, some conditions call for the use of Biofreeze or similar topical analgesic cream to relieve pain during massage.

3. Effleurage may be done with one or both hands.

4. Some techniques choose to use the tips of the fingers, whereas others advocate the use of the entire palm and fingers.

5. The movements are long, gentle and direct pressure toward the thorax.

a. For example, when providing effleurage to the lower leg the gliding pressure is heaviest at the distal end of the foot and becomes lighter as the hands move proximally on the leg.

6. At the end of the area being massaged, release all pressure, but keep your hands in constant contact with the skin and slide over the skin returning to the starting position.

a. This technique of effleurage is commonly called "Trees" or "Hearts" as this is the shape of effleurage massage being longitudinal from the distal position

to the proximal position and coming out and
around returning to the starting position.
C. *Shingles* is a method of "soft" massage where one stroke is
laid on top of the previous stroke like laying shingles on
a roof.
1.   This technique consists of placing the palm and fingers
of one hand on the area to be treated and moving the
hand toward you.
2.   As that hand is finishing the stroke, the other hand is
starting the next stroke.
3.   There is always hand contact with the patient.
4.   Often the hands move incrementally from a more distal
position to a more proximal position.
a.   For example, you may start shingle massage strokes
at the foot and gradually work proximally toward
the thigh.
b.   Remember to always pull the shingle massage
strokes toward the thorax or from distal to proximal
positions.
D. *Fulling* is another "soft" massage technique where the two
hands work from opposite sides and pull toward the middle.
1.   This technique is especially effective in the low back
region where the clinician can pull from right and left
sides toward the middle.
2.   This can also be effectively utilized in the extremities
where the clinician's hands would pull from outside and
inside positions toward the middle.
3.   It is especially important to realize that this technique
provides massage pressure perpendicular to the muscle
and connective tissues being treated.
E. *Swedish* is one more "soft" massage technique that actually
utilizes a progression from effleurage to shingles to fulling.
1.   Some Swedish techniques may also include Petrissage
and/or Tapotement ("hard") techniques as a fourth and
fifth levels of progression.
2.   It is important to realize the progressive techniques of
Swedish massage decrease the tactile accommodation of
just one massage technique.
a.   Tactile accommodation commonly occurs in the
body when your skin becomes accustomed to a particular object or pressure.

        b.   For example, when you first put your watch on your wrist it is noticeable to your consciousness. However, after a while it is barely perceptible unless moved or bumped. This is the process of tactile accommodation.

        c.   Tactile accommodation also occurs with single massage techniques which causes the patient to request harder massage treatment.

            i.   This can be a good thing if needing to release deep tissues.

            ii.   However, tactile accommodation can be a bad thing if the patient becomes numb and harder massage treatment actually injures soft tissue.

F.   *Petrissage* is a type of "hard" massage that involves kneading the muscles like a person would knead bread dough. The tissue is actually picked up and minimal or no lubricant is used in this technique.

    1.   This technique involves kneading tissues between the fingers of one hand and the Thenar eminence and thumb of the other hand.

    2.   Alternately, tissue may be picked up and compressed or rolled against bone or other dense tissue.

        a.   Normal repetitions of 7 to 10 petrissage kneading is performed in an area before moving to the next.

    3.   Small areas are normally worked and the progression is always done from distal positions toward proximal positions.

G.   *Knuckling* is another "hard" type of massage where a very deep stroke performed by making a fist and placing the dorsal surfaces of the first phalanges of the fingers on the area to be treated while the wrists are relaxed.

    1.   The stroke consists of forcefully extending the wrists in a flicking motion so the knuckles between the first and second phalanges provide the massage.

    2.   The direction of force is always from distal to proximal.

H.   *Shiatsu* "hard" massage is based on the Chinese theory of circulation and energy meridians running throughout the body.

    1.   This technique requires the patient's participation with the clinician in coordinating the breathing with massage treatments.

2.   Shiatsu is essentially a form of acupressure that is rhythmic and lasts from four to twelve seconds on specific meridian points using the fingers.

3.   No skin lubricant is used for this technique.

I.   *Myofascial Release* is a form of "hard" massage that is slow and involves manual stretching and twisting motions by the clinician.

1.   Originally developed by Cyriax and Barnes, Myofascial release is one of the only massage techniques that actually stretches and releases the fascia, (i.e., sheath covering muscle tissue).

2.   It is particularly efficacious in the cervical spine and for the diagnosis of fasciitis.

i.   Make sure you perform a Cervical Artery Sufficiency test and have a negative result before performing this massage technique in the neck.

3.   The distraction force is applied first.

4.   Then the twisting force is applied.

5.   Finally, the clinician's thumb(s) apply deep pressure over the stretched and twisted soft tissue.

6.   Each treatment progression is held for 30 seconds or more and often repeated more than 10 times.

J.   *Friction* massage is a "hard" technique where the skin is moved over the involved tissues with significant compression force and no lubricant.

1.   Friction massage is ALWAYS performed across, or perpendicular to muscle fibers.

2.   The anterior surface of the thumb and/or the Thenar eminence are the areas utilized by the clinician.

3.   The greatest pressure should be applied at the distal portion and lessened while moving proximally.

a.   Normal moderate to high speed repetitions of 7 to 10 friction massage strokes are performed in one specific area (usually a finger width wide) before moving to the next.

K.   *Tapotement* is a massage technique that involves one of seven types of percussion of the tissues:

1.   Raindrops are light percussion done with the finger tips as if using a typewriter or as if it were raining.

2. Tapping is done with the volar surface of the fingers keeping them extended and together while alternating hands in rapid succession.
3. Pincemont is done with a rapid and gentle pinching of the tissues between the thumbs and index fingers.
4. Slapping is done with the palms and fingers in extension and together while alternating hands in rapid succession.
5. Cupping is performed the same as slapping, only the hands are cupped.
6. Hacking is performed with the palms facing each other and the fingers relaxed. Use the ulnar borders of the hands and alternately and rapidly abduct and adduct the wrists without flexing and extending the elbows.
7. Beating is performed the same as hacking, but make a fist and use the ulnar borders of the fists.

APPENDICES

Appendix A:

ANATOMY/NEUROANATOMY
CHARTS [6,18,34,39,42,44,48,62,63,75,80,94106,115,149]

MUSCLES–HEAD & TRUNK

	ORIGIN	INSERTION	ACTION	NERVE
NECK-ANTERIOR				
PLATYSMA	CLAVICLE	MANDIBLE	DEPRESS JAW	CN-7 FACIAL
STERNOCLEIDO-MASTOID	MANUBRIUM/ ⅓ CLAVICLE	MASTOID PROCESS	FLEX OR ROTATE HEAD	CN-11 ACCESSORY
SUPRAHYOID GROUP	MASTOID PROCESS MANDIBLE	HYOID BONE	DEPRESS JAW	CN-5 AND 7 TRIGEMINAL/ FACIAL
ANTERIOR SCALENE	C3-6 TRANSVERSE PROCESSES	RIB #1	ELEVATE RIB & FLEX NECK	C5-7
MIDDLE SCALENE	C2-7 TRANSVERSE PROCESSES	RIB #1	ELEVATE RIB & FLEX NECK	C3-8
POSTERIOR SCALENE	C5-7 TRANSVERSE PROCESSES	RIB #2	ELEVATE RIB & FLEX NECK	C7-8
LONGUS CAPITIS	C3-6 TRANSVERSE PROCESSES	OCCIPITAL BONE	FLEX OR ROTATE HEAD	C1-4
LONGUS COLI	C3-T3 TRANSVERSE PROCESSES	ATLAS BONE & C2-6 VERTEBRAE	FLEX OR ROTATE HEAD	C2-6
NECK/BACK				
SPLENIUS CAPITIS	C1-6 SPINOUS PROCESSES	MASTOID PROCESS	SIDE BEND OR ROTATE OR EXTEND HEAD	DORSAL PRIMARY RAMI
ERECTOR SPINAE GROUP	RIBS #1-12	TRANSVERSE AND SPINOUS	ROTATE OR EXTEND HEAD	DORSAL PRIMARY RAMI
TRANSVERSI-SPINALIS GROUP	TRANSVERSE PROCESSES C1-L5	SPINOUS PROCESSES	ROTATE OR EXTEND SPINE	DORSAL PRIMARY RAMI
SUBOCCIPITAL TRIANGLE GROUP	ATLAS & AXIS	OCCIPITAL BONE	SIDE BEND OR ROTATE OR EXTEND HEAD	C1 SUBOCCIPITAL
TRAPEZIUS	OCCIPUT TO SPINOUS PROCESSES C7-	ACROMION & SCAPULAR SPINE	SCAPULAR RETRACTION, ROTATION,	CN-11 ACCESSORY

(continued)

MUSCLES–HEAD & TRUNK (*continued*)

	ORIGIN	INSERTION	ACTION	NERVE
NECK/BACK (*continued*)				
LEVATOR SCAPULAE	TRANSVERSE PROCESSES C1-4	SUPERIOR/ MED. SCAPULAR BORDER	SCAPULAR ELEVATION	DORSAL SCAPULAR C-5
RHOMBOID MINOR	SPINOUS PROCESSES C7-T1	SCAPULAR SPINE	SCAPULAR RETRACTION	DORSAL SCAPULAR C-5
RHOMBOID MAJOR	SPINOUS PROCESSES T2-5	INFERIOR/ MED. SCAPULAR BORDER	SCAPULAR RETRACTION	DORSAL SCAPULAR C-5
SERRATUS POSTERIOR	SPINOUS PROCESSES C7-L3	RIBS #2-12	SUPERIOR FIBERS ELEVATE RIBS	INTERCOSTAL T1-12
ABDOMEN				
EXTERNAL INTERCOSTALS	INFERIOR RIBS #1-12	SUPERIOR RIB CAUDAL TO ORIGIN	ELEVATE RIBS	INTERCOSTAL T1-12
INTERNAL INTERCOSTALS	INFERIOR RIBS #1-12	SUPERIOR RIB	DEPRESS RIBS	INTERCOSTAL T1-12
EXTERNAL OBLIQUE	RIBS #4-12	ILIAC CREST	FLEX OR SIDE BEND OR TRUNK	INTERCOSTAL T7-12
INTERNAL OBLIQUE	ILIAC CREST	RIBS #9-12	FLEX OR SIDE BEND TRUNK	INTERCOSTAL T7-12
TRANSVERSUS ABDOMINIS	RIBS #6-12	LINEA ALBA	COMPRESS ABDOMEN	INTERCOSTAL T7-12
RECTUS ABDOMINIS	PUBIC CREST	COSTAL CARTILAGE 5-7	FLEX TRUNK, DEPRESS RIBS	INTERCOSTAL T7-12
PYRAMIDALIS	PUBIC BODY	LINEA ALBA	TENSES LINEA ALBA	SUBCOSTAL T12
JAW				
TEMPORALIS	TEMPORAL FOSSA	RAMUS OF MANDIBLE	ELEVATE & RETRACT MANDIBLE	CN-5 TRIGEMINAL
MASSETER	ZYGOMATIC ARCH	RAMUS OF MANDIBLE	ELEVATE MANDIBLE	CN-5 TRIGEMINAL
LATERAL PTERYGOID	SPHENOID & LATERAL PTERYGOID	TMJ DISC AND NECK OF MANDIBLE	PROTRACT & DEPRESS MANDIBLE	CN-5 TRIGEMINAL
MEDIAL PTERYGOID	MEDIAL PTERYGOID PLATE	MEDIAL ANGLE & RAMUS OF MANDIBLE	PROTRACT & ELEVATE MANDIBLE	CN-5 TRIGEMINAL
EYE				
SUPERIOR RECTUS	COMMON TENDINOUS RING	SCLERA	SUPERIOR/ LATERAL EYE MOVEMENT	CN-3 OCULOMOTOR
INFERIOR RECTUS	COMMON TENDINOUS RING	SCLERA	INFERIOR/ LATERAL EYE MOVEMENT	CN-3 OCULOMOTOR

	ORIGIN	INSERTION	ACTION	NERVE
MEDIAL RECTUS	COMMON TENDINOUS RING	SCLERA	MEDIAL EYE MOVEMENT	CN-3 OCULOMOTOR
LATERAL RECTUS	COMMON TENDINOUS RING	SCLERA	LATERAL EYE MOVEMENT	CN-6 ABDUCENS
SUPERIOR OBLIQUE	SPHENOID BONE	SCLERA	INFERIOR/ MEDIAL EYE MOVEMENT	CN-4 TROCHLEAR
INFERIOR OBLIQUE	FLOOR OF ORBIT	SCLERA	SUPERIOR/ MEDIAL EYE MOVEMENT	CN-3 OCULOMOTOR

MUSCLES–UPPER EXTREMITY

	ORIGIN	INSERTION	ACTION	NERVE
UPPER EXTREMITY				
PECTORALIS MAJOR	CLAVICLE & MANUBRIUM	LATERAL BICIPITAL	DEPRESS, FLEX, ADDUCT AND INTERNAL ROTATE	MEDIAL & LATERAL PECTORAL C5-T1
PECTORALIS MINOR	RIBS #2-5	CORACOID PROCESS	DEPRESS SHOULDER	MEDIAL PECTORAL C8-T1
SUBCLAVIUS	RIB #1 & MANUBRIUM	INFERIOR CLAVICLE	DEPRESS CLAVICLE	NERVE TO SUBCLAVIUS C5
SERRATUS ANTERIOR	RIBS #1-8	MEDIAL SCAPULAR BORDER	PROTRACTS AND ROTATES SCAPULA	LONG THORACIC C5-7
DELTOID	CLAVICLE, ACROMION & SCAPULA	DELTOID TUBEROSITY	FLEX, EXTEND, INTERNAL ROTATE, ABDUCT, ADDUCT	AXILLARY C6-7
SUPRASPINATUS	SUPRASPINOUS FOSSA	GREATER TUBERCLE	ABDUCTS SHOULDER	SUPRA-SCAPULAR C5-6
INFRASPINATUS	INFRASPINOUS FOSSA	GREATER TUBERCLE	EXTERNAL ROTATES SHOULDER	SUPRA-SCAPULAR C5-6
SUBSCAPULARIS	SUBSCAPULAR FOSSA	LESSER TUBERCLE	INTERNAL ROTATES SHOULDER	UPPER & LOWER SUBSCAPULAR C5-6
TERES MINOR	SUPERIOR LATERAL SCAPULAR BORDER	GREATER TUBERCLE	EXTERNAL ROTATES SHOULDER	AXILLARY C6-7
TERES MAJOR	INFERIOR SCAPULAR ANGLE	MEDIAL BICIPITAL GROOVE	INTERNAL ROTATES & ADDUCTS SHOULDER	LOWER SUBSCAPULAR C5-6

(*continued*)

MUSCLES–UPPER EXTREMITY (*continued*)

	ORIGIN	INSERTION	ACTION	NERVE
UPPER EXTREMITY (*continued*)				
LATISSIMUS DORSI	SPINOUS PROCESSES T7-12, ILIAC CREST	INFERIOR BICIPITAL GROOVE	INTERNAL ROTATES & ADDUCTS SHOULDER	THORACO-DORSAL C7-8
CORACO-BRACHIALIS	CORACOID PROCESS	MEDIAL MID HUMERUS	FLEXES & ADDUCTS SHOULDER	MUSCULO-CUTANEOUS C5-7
BICEPS BRACHI				
LONG HEAD	SUPRAGLENOID TUBERCLE	RADIAL TUBEROSITY	FLEXES & SUPINATES FOREARM	MUSCULO-CUTANEOUS C5-7
SHORT HEAD	CORACOID PROCESS	RADIAL TUBEROSITY	FLEXES & SUPINATES FOREARM	MUSCULO-CUTANEOUS C5-7
BRACHIALIS	INFERIOR ANTERIOR HUMERUS	ULNAR TUBEROSITY	FLEXES FOREARM	MUSCULO-CUTANEOUS C5-7
TRICEPS				
LONG HEAD	INFRAGLENOID TUBERCLE	OLECRANON	EXTENDS FOREARM	RADIAL C5-T1
LATERAL HEAD	SUPERIOR RADIAL GROOVE	OLECRANON	EXTENDS FOREARM	RADIAL C5-T1
MEDIAL HEAD	INFERIOR RADIAL GROOVE	OLECRANON	EXTENDS FOREARM	RADIAL C5-T1
ANCONEUS	LATERAL EPICONDYLE	OLECRANON & POSTERIOR ULNA	EXTENDS FOREARM	RADIAL C5-T1
PRONATOR TERES	MEDIAL EPICONDYLE & CORONOID PROCESS ULNA	MID LATERAL RADIUS	PRONATES FOREARM	MEDIAN C5-T1
FLEXOR CARPI RADIALIS	MEDIAL EPICONDYLE	METACARPALS #2-3	FLEXES FOREARM & WRIST + ABDUCT WRIST	MEDIAN C5-T1
PALMARIS LONGUS	MEDIAL EPICONDYLE	FLEXOR RETINACULUM	FLEXES FOREARM & WRIST	MEDIAN C5-T1
FLEXOR CARPI ULNARIS	MEDIAL EPICONDYLE & OLECRANON	PISIFORM, HOOK OF HAMATE & METACARPAL #5	FLEXES FOREARM & WRIST + ADDUCT WRIST	ULNAR C7-T1
FLEXOR DIGITORUM SUPERFICIALIS	MEDIAL EPICONDYLE & ULNA/ RADIAL SURFACES	MID PHALANX #2-5	FLEXES FOREARM & WRIST + PIP JOINT	MEDIAN C5-T1
FLEXOR DIGITORUM PROFUNDUS	ANTERIOR/ MEDIAL ULNA & INTEROSSEUS MEMBRANE	DISTAL PHALANX #2-5	FLEXES WRIST & DIP JOINT	ULNAR & MEDIAN C5-T1

	ORIGIN	INSERTION	ACTION	NERVE
FLEXOR POLLICIS LONGUS	INTEROSSEUS MEMBRANE & ULNA/ RADIAL SURFACES	DISTAL PHALANX #1	FLEXES THUMB	MEDIAN C5-T1
PRONATOR QUADRATUS	ANTERIOR/ DISTAL ULNA	ANTERIOR/ DISTAL RADIUS	PRONATES FOREARM	MEDIAN C5-T1
BRACHIORADIALIS	LATERAL SUPRA-CONDYLAR RIDGE	RADIAL STYLOID PROCESS	FLEXES FOREARM	RADIAL C5-T1
EXTENSOR CARPI RADIALIS LONGUS	LATERAL SUPRA-CONDYLAR RIDGE	METACARPAL #2	EXTENDS AND ABDUCTS WRIST	RADIAL C5-T1
EXTENSOR CARPI RADIALIS BREVIS	LATERAL EPICONDYLE	METACARPAL #3	EXTENDS AND ABDUCTS WRIST	RADIAL C5-T1
EXTENSOR DIGITORUM	LATERAL EPICONDYLE	PIP AND MID PHALANX #2-5	EXTENDS FINGERS & WRIST	RADIAL C5-T1
EXTENSOR I DIGITI MINIM	COMMON EXTENSOR	MID PHALANX AND DIP #5	EXTENDS FINGER #5	RADIAL C5-T1
EXTENSOR CARPI ULNARIS	LATERAL EPICONDYLE & ULNA	METACARPAL #5	EXTENDS & ADDUCTS WRIST	RADIAL C5-T1
SUPINATOR	LATERAL EPICONDYLE & RADIUS	LATERAL PROXIMAL RADIUS	SUPINATES FOREARM	RADIAL C5-T1
ABDUCTOR POLLICIS LONGUS	INTEROSSEUS MEMBRANE & POSTERIOR RADIUS & ULNA	METACARPAL #1	ABDUCTS THUMB AND WRIST	RADIAL C5-T1
EXTENSOR POLLICIS LONGUS	INTEROSSEUS MEMBRANE & POSTERIOR ULNA	DIP #1	EXTENDS THUMB & ABDUCTS WRIST	RADIAL C5-T1
EXTENSOR POLLICIS BREVIS	INTEROSSEUS MEMBRANE & POSTERIOR RADIUS	PIP #1	EXTENDS PROXIMAL PHALANX AND ABDUCTS WRIST	RADIAL C5-T1
EXTENSOR INDICIS	INTEROSSEUS MEMBRANE & POSTERIOR ULNA	DISTAL PHALANX #2	EXTENDS INDEX FINGER	RADIAL C5-T1
HAND INTRINSICS				
ABDUCTOR POLLICIS BREVIS	FLEXOR RETINACULUM, SCAPHOID, TRAPEZIUM	PROXIMAL PHALANX #1	ABDUCTS THUMB	MEDIAN C5-T1
FLEXOR POLLICIS BREVIS	FLEXOR RETINACULUM, TRAPEZIUM	PROXIMAL PHALANX #1	FLEXES THUMB	MEDIAN C5-T1
OPPONENS POLLICIS	FLEXOR RETINACULUM, TRAPEZIUM	METACARPAL #1	OPPOSITION THUMB	MEDIAN C5-T1
LUMBRICALS (4)	LATERAL FLEXOR DIGITORUM PROFUNDUS TENDONS	LATERAL EXTENSOR EXPANSION	FLEXES MCP #2-5 & EXTENDS DIP/PIP #2-5	MEDIAN & ULNAR C5-T1

(*continued*)

MUSCLES–UPPER EXTREMITY (*continued*)

	ORIGIN	INSERTION	ACTION	NERVE
HAND INTRINSICS (*continued*)				
DORSAL INTEROSSEI (4)	METACARPALS	LATERAL PROXIMAL PHALANX #2-5	ABDUCTS FINGERS	ULNAR C7-T1
PALMER INTEROSSEI (3)	METACARPALS	PROXIMAL PHALANX	ADDUCTS FINGERS	ULNAR C7-T1
ADDUCTOR POLLICIS	CAPITATE, METACARPALS #2-3	PROXIMAL PHALANX #1	ADDUCTS THUMB	ULNAR C7-T1
ABDUCTOR DIGITI MINIMI	PISIFORM	MEDIAL PROXIMAL PHALANX #5	ABDUCTS FINGER #5	ULNAR C7-T1
FLEXOR DIGITI MINIMI BREVIS	HOOK OF HAMATE	MEDIAL PROXIMAL PHALANX #5	FLEXES FINGER #5	ULNAR C7-T1
OPPONENS DIGITI MINIMI	HOOK OF HAMATE	MEDIAL METACARPAL	OPPOSITION FINGER #5	ULNAR C7-T1

Anatomy of Hand/Finger Flexors

Zone 1–from insertion of Profundus tendon at distal phalanx to distal insertion of Sublimis

Zone 2–Bunnell's "no man's land" between insertion of Sublimis and distal palmer crease

Zone 3–"Area of Lumbrical Origin" from A1 pulleys to distal margin of Transverse Carpal ligament

Zone 4–Area covered by transverse carpal ligament

Zone 5–Area proximal to transverse carpal ligament

Anatomy of Hand/Finger Extensors

Zone	Finger	Thumb
1	DIP joint	IP joint
2	Mid Phalanx	Proximal Phalanx
3	Apex of PIP joint	MCP joint
4	Proximal Phalanx	Metacarpal
5	Apex of MCP joint	
6	Dorsal Hand	
7	Dorsal Retinaculum	Dorsal Retinaculum
8	Distal Forearm	Distal Forearm

MUSCLES–LOWER EXTREMITY

	ORIGIN	INSERTION	ACTION	NERVE
LOWER EXTREMITY				
ILIOPSOAS	TRANSVERSE PROCESSES T12-L5	LESSER TROCHANTER	FLEXES HIP	L2-3
PSOAS MINOR	VERTEBRAL BODY T12-L1	PECTINEAL LINE	FLEXES HIP	L1
QUADRATUS LUMBORUM	ILIAC CREST L3-5	RIB #12, L1-3	SIDE BENDS TRUNK	T12-L
PIRIFORMIS	SACRUM	GREATER TROCHANTER	EXTERNAL ROTATES HIP & ABDUCTS HIP	S1-2
PELVIC EXTERNAL ROTATOR GROUP	ISCHIUM	GREATER TROCHANTER	EXTERNAL ROTATES HIP	L4-S2
GLUTEUS MAXIMUS	PSIS	ILIO TIBIAL BAND	EXTERNAL ROT., EXTENDS & ABDUCTS HIP	INFERIOR GLUTEAL L5-S2
SARTORIUS	ASIS	PES ANSERINUS	FLEXES, ABDUCTS, EXTERNAL ROT.	FEMORAL L2-4
RECTUS FEMORIS	ASIS	TIBIAL TUBEROSITY	FLEXES HIP & EXTENDS KNEE	FEMORAL L2-4
VASTUS LATERALIS	LATERAL LINEA ASPERA	TIBIAL TUBEROSITY	EXTENDS KNEE	FEMORAL L2-4
VASTUS MEDIALIS	MEDIAL LINEA ASPERA	TIBIAL TUBEROSITY	EXTENDS KNEE	FEMORAL L2-4
VASTUS INTERMEDIUS	ANTERIOR FEMUR	QUADRICEPS TENDON	EXTENDS KNEE	FEMORAL L2-4
ARTICULARIS GENU	ANTERIOR FEMUR	SUPERIOR KNEE JOINT CAPSULE	ELEVATES CAPSULE IN EXTENSION	FEMORAL L2-4
GRACILIS	INFERIOR PUBIC RAMUS	PES ANSERINUS	FLEXES, INTERNAL ROT., ADDUCTS HIP	OBTURATOR L3-4
PECTINEUS	PECTIN OF PUBIS	PECTINEAL LINE	FLEXES, INTERNAL ROT., ADDUCTS HIP	FEMORAL L2-4
ADDUCTOR LONGUS	SUPERIOR PUBIC RAMUS	MEDIAL LINEA ASPERA	FLEXES, INTERNAL ROT., ADDUCTS HIP	OBTURATOR L3-4
ADDUCTOR BREVIS	INFERIOR PUBIC RAMUS	PECTINEAL LINE	FLEXES, INTERNAL ROT., ADDUCTS HIP	ANTERIOR OBTURATOR L3-4
ADDUCTOR MAGNUS	ISCHIOPUBIC RAMUS & ISCHIAL TUBEROSITY	LINEA ASPERA & ADDUCTOR TUBERCLE	EXTENDS, INTERNAL ROT., ADDUCTS HIP	POSTERIOR OBTURATOR & TIBIAL SCIATIC L3-S2
GLUTEUS MEDIUS	MID GLUTEAL LINE	GREATER TROCHANTER	INTERNAL ROTATES, ABDUCTS HIP	SUPERIOR GLUTEAL L4-S1

(*continued*)

MUSCLES–LOWER EXTREMITY (*continued*)

	ORIGIN	INSERTION	ACTION	NERVE
LOWER EXTREMITY (*continued*)				
GLUTEUS MINIMUS	MID INFERIOR GLUTEAL LINE	GREATER TROCHANTER	INTERNAL ROTATES, ABDUCTS HIP	SUPERIOR GLUTEAL L4-S1
TENSOR FASCIA LATAE	EXTERNAL ILIAC CREST	ILIOTIBIAL BAND	INTERNAL ROTATES, FLEXES, ABDUCTS	SUPERIOR GLUTEAL L4-S1
SEMITENDINOSUS	ISCHIAL TUBEROSITY	PES ANSERINUS	FLEXES KNEE, INTERNAL ROT., AND EXTENDS HIP	TIBIAL-SCIATIC L5-S2
SEMI-MEMBRANOSUS	ISCHIAL TUBEROSITY	POSTERIOR TIBIA	FLEXES KNEE, INTERNAL ROT., AND EXTENDS HIP	TIBIAL-SCIATIC L5-S2
BICEPS FEMORIS				
LONG HEAD	ISCHIAL TUBEROSITY	FIBULA	EXTENDS HIP	TIBIAL-SCIATIC L5-S2
SHORT HEAD	LATERAL LINEA ASPERA	FIBULA	FLEXES KNEE, EXTERNAL ROTATES HIP	COMMON FIBULAR-SCIATIC L5-S2
TIBIALIS ANTERIOR	LATERAL TIBIAL CONDYLE	MEDIAL CUNEIFORM & METATARSAL #1	DORSIFLEXES & INVERTS ANKLE	DEEP FIBULAR L4-S1
EXTENSOR HALLUCIS LONGUS	MID FIBULA	DIP GREAT TOE	DORSIFLEXES & INVERTS ANKLE + EXTENDS TOE #1	DEEP FIBULAR L4-S1
EXTENSOR DIGITORUM LONGUS	LATERAL TIBIAL CONDYLE & ANTERIOR FIBULA	EXTENSOR EXPANSION TOES #2-5	DORSIFLEXES ANKLE + EXTENDS TOES #2-5	DEEP FIBULAR L4-S1
EXTENSOR HALLUCIS BREVIS	LATERAL CALCANEUS	PIP GREAT TOE	EXTENDS TOE #1	DEEP FIBULAR L4-S1
EXTENSOR DIGITORUM BREVIS	LATERAL CALCANEUS	EXTENSOR EXPANSION TOES #2-4	EXTENDS TOES #2-4	DEEP FIBULAR L4-S1
FIBULARIS LONGUS	UPPER ⅔ LATERAL FIBULA	MEDIAL CUNEIFORM & METATARSAL #1	PLANTARFLEX, EVERTS AND ABDUCTS ANKLE	SUPERFICIAL FIBULAR
FIBULARIS BREVIS	LOWER ⅔ LATERAL FIBULA	METATARSAL #5	PLANTARFLEX, EVERTS AND ABDUCTS ANKLE	SUPERFICIAL FIBULAR
GASTROCNEMIUS	MEDIAL & LATERAL FEMORAL CONDYLES	CALCANEUS	PLANTARFLEX ANKLE AND FLEX KNEE	TIBIAL
PLANTARIS	LATERAL SUPRA-CONDYLAR FEMUR	CALCANEAL TENDON	PLANTARFLEX ANKLE AND FLEX KNEE	TIBIAL

	ORIGIN	INSERTION	ACTION	NERVE
SOLEUS	POSTERIOR FIBULA & SOLEAL LINE	CALCANEUS	PLANTARFLEX ANKLE	TIBIAL
POPLITEUS	LATERAL FEMORAL CONDYLE	TIBIAL CREST	FLEXES KNEE & INTERNAL ROTATES TIBIA	TIBIAL
TIBIALIS POSTERIOR	TIB/FIB INTEROSSEUS MEMBRANE	CUNEIFORMS, NAVICULAR & METATARSALS	PLANTARFLEX AND SUPINATE ANKLE	TIBIAL
FLEXOR DIGITORUM LONGUS	TIBIA, BELOW SOLEAL LINE	DIP #2-4	PLANTARFLEX & SUPINATE ANKLE + FLEX TOES #2-4	TIBIAL
FLEXOR HALLUCIS LONGUS	POSTERIOR FIBULA	DIP #1	PLANTARFLEX & SUPINATE ANKLE + FLEX TOE #1	TIBIAL
FOOT INTRINSICS				
ABDUCTOR HALLUCIS	CALCANEUS	PROXIMAL PHALANX	ABDUCTS GREAT TOE	MEDIAL PLANTAR L4-5
FLEXOR HALLUCIS BREVIS	CUBOID, CUNEIFORM #3	PROXIMAL PHALANX #1	FLEXES GREAT TOE	MEDIAL PLANTAR L4-5
FLEXOR DIGITORUM BREVIS	CALCANEUS	MID PHALANX #2-5	FLEXES TOES #2-5	MEDIAL PLANTAR L4-5
LUMBRICAL (1)	FLEXOR DIGITORUM LONGUS TENDONS	PIP EXTENSOR EXPANSION	FLEXES MTP JOINT AND EXTENDS IP JOINT	MEDIAL PLANTAR L4-5
ABDUCTOR DIGITI MINIMI	CALCANEUS	PROXIMAL PHALANX	ABDUCTS TOE #5	LATERAL PLANTAR S1-2
FLEXOR DIGITI MINIMI BREVIS	METATARSAL #5	PROXIMAL PHALANX	FLEXES TOE #5	LATERAL PLANTAR S1-2
QUADRATUS PLANTAE	CALCANEUS	FLEXOR DIGITORUM LONGUS	FLEXES TOES #2-5	LATERAL PLANTAR S1-2
LUMBRICALS (3)	FLEXOR DIGITORUM LONGUS TENDONS	PROX. PHALANX & EXTENSOR EXPANSION	FLEXES MTP AND EXTENDS IP JOINTS #2-5	LATERAL PLANTAR S1-2
ADDUCTOR HALLUCIS	METATARSALS #2-4	PROXIMAL PHALANX #1	ADDUCTS GREAT TOE	LATERAL PLANTAR S1-2
PLANTAR INTEROSSEI (3)	METATARSALS #3-5	PROXIMAL PHALANX	ADDUCTS TOES	LATERAL PLANTAR S1-2
DORSAL INTEROSSEI (4)	METATARSAL SHAFTS #2-5	PROXIMAL PHALANX	ABDUCTS TOES	LATERAL PLANTAR S1-2

LIGAMENTS

LOCATION	NAME	RESTRICTS
SHOULDER		
AC JOINT	SUPERIOR/ INFERIOR ACROMIO-CLAVICULAR LIGAMENTS	CAPSULE SEPARATION
	CORACOCLAVICULAR	SUPERIOR CLAVICLE DISPLACEMENT
GLENOHUMERAL JOINT	CORACOHUMERAL	EXTERNAL ROTATION + GRAVITY
	GLENOHUMERAL	EXTERNAL ROTATION + FLEXION
	CORACOACROMIAL	SUPERIOR HUMERAL DISPLACEMENT
ELBOW		
HUMERO-ULNAR JOINT	ULNAR COLLATERAL	VALGUS STRESS
HUMERO-RADIAL JOINT	RADIAL COLLATERAL	VARUS STRESS
PROXIMAL RADIO-ULNAR JOINT	ANNULAR	RADIAL HEAD DISLOCATION
DISTAL RADIO-ULNAR JOINT	INTEROSSEUS MEMBRANE	RADIUS & ULNAR SEPARATION
WRIST		
RADIO-CARPAL JOINT	RADIAL COLLATERAL	VARUS STRESS
	ULNAR COLLATERAL	VALGUS STRESS
	DORSAL RADIOCARPAL	DORSAL STRESS & JOINT SEPARATION
	PALMER RADIOCARPAL	VOLAR STRESS & JOINT SEPARATION
HIP		
FEMORAL-PELVIC JOINT	ILIOFEMORAL	ADDUCTION, EXTENSION AND ABDUCTION STRESS
	PUBOFEMORAL	ABDUCTION AND EXTENSION STRESS
	ISCHIOFEMORAL	INTERNAL ROTATION & EXTENSION STRESS
	ZONA ORBICULARIS	JOINT SEPARATION
KNEE		
TIBIAL-FEMORAL JOINT	MEDIAL COLLATERAL	VALGUS STRESS
	LATERAL COLLATERAL	VARUS STRESS
	ANTERIOR CRUCIATE	EXTENSION
	POSTERIOR CRUCIATE	FLEXION
ANKLE		
TALOCRURAL JOINT	DELTOID	VALGUS STRESS
	LATERAL COLLATERAL	VARUS STRESS

NEUROANATOMY

I. **MYOTOMAL** testing against manual resistance and noting asymmetrical findings:
   A. C1- cervical flexion.
   B. C2- cervical extension.
   C. C3- cervical sidebending or rotation.
   D. C4- shoulder shrug up (Trapezius, Levator Scapula).
   E. C5- shoulder abduction (Deltoid).
   F. C6- elbow flexion (Biceps, Brachialis).
   G. C7- elbow extension (Triceps, Anconeus).
   H. C8- thumb extension.
   I. T1- finger abduction.
   J. T12-L2 hip flexion (Iliopsoas, Rectus Femoris).
   K. L2-4 knee extension (Quadriceps).
   L. L4 ankle dorsiflexion (Tibialis Anterior).
   M. L5 great toe extension (Extensor Hallucis Longus).
   N. S1-2 ankle plantarflexion (Gastrocnemius)

II. **DERMATOMAL** testing for light touch/deep pressure or sharp/dull or hot/cold and noting symmetrical findings:
   A. C1- face (forehead).
   B. C2- face (cheek).
   C. C3- face (chin).
   D. C4- upper Trapezius.
   E. C5- deltoid.
   F. C6- thumb.
   G. C7- fingers #3-4.
   H. C8- finger #5.
   I. T1- ulnar surface.
   J. L1- ASIS.
   K. L2- anterior lateral thigh.
   L. L3- medial femoral condyle.
   M. L4- medial malleolus/great toe.
   N. L5- toes #2-4.
   O. S1- lateral malleolus/toe #5.
   P. S2- posterior lateral calf .
   Q. S3-5 ask patient regarding change in bowel/bladder function.

III. **SUPERFICIAL SENSORY NERVES** testing for light touch/deep pressure or sharp/dull or hot/cold and note asymmetrical findings:
   A. Most Commonly Involved Nerves:
       1. Axillary.
       2. Medial/Lateral Antebrachial Cutaneous.
       3. Radial.
       4. Median.
       5. Ulnar.
       6. Lateral/ Anterior/ Posterior Femoral Cutaneous.
       7. Saphenous.
       8. Common Fibular.
       9. Superficial Fibular.
       10. Deep Fibular.
       11. Sural.

IV. **SENSORY GLOVE-STOCKING PATTERN** testing for light touch/deep pressure or sharp/dull or hot/cold and noting asymmetrical findings:
   A. Most commonly affects hands or feet.
   B. Common causes include:
       1. Vascular problems.
       2. Toxins.
       3. Alcohol.
       4. Diabetes.

V. **DEEP TENDON REFLEX TESTING:**
   A. Biceps Tendon- C-5.
   B. Brachioradialis Tendon- C-6.
   C. Triceps- C-7.
   D. Patellar Tendon- L2.
   E. Achilles Tendon- S1.

VI. **CRANIAL NERVE TESTING**   **PRIMARY ACTION**

A.	CN 1 Olfactory	Smell
B.	CN 2 Optic	Vision
C.	CN 3 Oculomotor	Eye movement
D.	CN 4 Trochlear	Eye movement
E.	CN 5 Trigeminal	Muscles of mastication
F.	CN 6 Abducens	Eye movement
G.	CN 7 Facial	Facial muscles
H.	CN 8 Vestibulocochlear	Hearing & Equilibrium
I.	CN 9 Glossopharyngeal	Swallowing & Taste

J. CN 10 Vagus   Respiration/Heart rate
K. CN 11 Accessory   Trapezius
L. CN 12 Hypoglossal   Muscles of the tongue

VII. **ANATOMICAL CLINICAL RELEVANCE:**

A. Remember all action/motions are listed in the anatomical plane with the palms supinated.

B. The most unstable joint in the body is the shoulder joint.

C. The most stable joint in the body is the hip joint.

D. Muscles that comprise the rotator cuff include:
    1. Supraspinatus.
    2. Infraspinatus.
    3. Subscapularis.
    4. Teres Minor.

E. Muscles that comprise the Pes Anserinus include:
    1. Semitendinosus.
    2. Gracilis.
    3. Sartorius.

F. Muscles that comprise the pelvic external rotator group include:
    1. Obturator Internus.
    2. Superior Gemelles.
    3. Inferior Gemelles.
    4. Quadratus Femoris.
    5. Obturator Externus.

G. Muscles that comprise the Erector Spinae group include:
    1. Iliocostalis.
    2. Longissimus.
    3. Spinalis.

H. Muscles that comprise the Transversospinalis group include:
    1. Semispinalis.
    2. Multifidus.
    3. Rotatores.

I. Muscles that comprise the suboccipital triangle group include:
    1. Rectus Capitis.
    2. Posterior Major.
    3. Rectus Capitis Posterior Minor.
    4. Obliquous Capitis Superior.
    5. Obliquous Capitis Inferior.

J. Semispinalis Capitis and Cervicus muscles constitute the bulk of posterior neck muscle mass.
K. The Piriformis muscle is a dual action muscle:
    1. Below 90 degrees hip flexion the muscle acts as an external rotator of the hip.
    2. Above 90 degrees hip flexion the muscle acts as a hip abductor.
L. The quadriceps group is comprised of the following:
    1. Rectus Femoris.
    2. Vastus Lateralis.
    3. Vastus Medialis.
    4. Vastus Intermedius.
M. Thumb motions are referred to at a 90 degree rotation of finger motions:
    1. Thumb abduction is in the finger flexion plane of motion.
    2. Thumb adduction is in the finger extension plane of motion.
    3. Thumb flexion is in the finger adduction plane of motion.
    4. Thumb extension is in the finger abduction plane of motion.
N. The Thenar Eminence consists of the following:
    1. Abductor Pollicis Brevis.
    2. Flexor Pollicis Brevis.
    3. Opponens Pollicis.
O. The Hypothenar Eminence consists of the following:
    1. Abductor Digiti Minimi.
    2. Flexor Digiti Minimi Brevis.
    3. Opponens Digiti Minimi.
P. The Suprahyoid group consists of the following:
    1. Digastric.
    2. Mylohyoid.
Q. The Infrahyoid group consists of the following:
    1. Sternohyoid.
    2. Sternothyroid.
    3. Thyrohyoid.
    4. Omohyoid.
R. The brachial plexus passes between the Anterior Scalene and Middle Scalene muscles.

S. A common site of pain in patients with rotator cuff strains includes the Deltoid insertion.
    1. This site is not referred pain, but an actual muscle strain in most cases and needs appropriate treatment in addition to the rotator cuff muscles involved.

Appendix B:

RANGE OF MOTION
CHART[6,18,34,39,42,44,48,62,63,75,80,94106,115,149]

RANGE OF MOTION

RIGHT		NORMAL	LEFT	
PROM	AROM		PROM	AROM
		NECK FLEXION 45 DEG		
		NECK EXTENSION 45 DEG		
		NECK ROTATION 60 DEG		
		NECK SIDEBENDING 45 DEG		
		TRUNK FLEXION 80 DEG		
		TRUNK EXTENSION 25 DEG		
		TRUNK ROTATION 45 DEG		
		TRUNK SIDEBENDING 35 DEG		
		SHOULDER FLEXION 180 DEG		
		SHOULDER EXTENSION 45 DEG		
		SHOULDER ABDUCTION 180 DEG		
		SHOULDER ADDUCTION 0 DEG		
		SHOULDER INTERNAL ROTATION 70 DEG		
		SHOULDER EXTERNAL ROTATION 90 DEG		
		ELBOW FLEXION 145 DEG		
		ELBOW EXTENSION 0 DEG		
		FOREARM SUPINATION 90 DEG		
		FOREARM PRONATION 90 DEG		
		WRIST FLEXION 80 DEG		
		WRIST EXTENSION 70 DEG		
		WRIST ULNAR DEVIATION 30 DEG		
		WRIST RADIAL DEVIATION 20 DEG		
		THUMB FLEXION (CMC) 0 DEG		
		THUMB EXTENSION (CMC) 45 DEG		
		THUMB ABDUCTION (CMC) 35 DEG		
		THUMB ADDUCTION (CMC) 0 DEG		
		THUMB FLEXION (MCP) 50 DEG		

348

RIGHT		NORMAL	LEFT	
PROM	AROM		PROM	AROM
		THUMB EXTENSION (MCP) 0 DEG		
		THUMB FLEXION (IP) 80 DEG		
		THUMB EXTENSION (IP) 0 DEG		
		INDEX FINGER FLEXION (MCP) 90 DEG		
		INDEX FINGER EXTENSION (MCP) 45 DEG		
		INDEX FINGER FLEXION (PIP) 100 DEG		
		INDEX FINGER EXTENSION (PIP) 0 DEG		
		INDEX FINGER FLEXION (DIP) 90 DEG		
		INDEX FINGER EXTENSION (DIP) 0 DEG		
		MIDDLE FINGER FLEXION (MCP) 90 DEG		
		MIDDLE FINGER EXTENSION (MCP) 45 DEG		
		MIDDLE FINGER FLEXION (PIP) 100 DEG		
		MIDDLE FINGER EXTENSION (PIP) 0 DEG		
		MIDDLE FINGER FLEXION (DIP) 90 DEG		
		MIDDLE FINGER EXTENSION (DIP) 0 DEG		
		RING FINGER FLEXION (MCP) 90 DEG		
		RING FINGER EXTENSION (MCP) 45 DEG		
		RING FINGER FLEXION (PIP) 100 DEG		
		RING FINGER EXTENSION (PIP) 0 DEG		
		RING FINGER FLEXION (DIP) 90 DEG		
		RING FINGER EXTENSION (DIP) 0 DEG		
		FIFTH FINGER FLEXION (MCP) 90 DEG		
		FIFTH FINGER EXTENSION (MCP) 45 DEG		
		FIFTH FINGER FLEXION (PIP) 90 DEG		
		FIFTH FINGER EXTENSION (PIP) 0 DEG		
		FIFTH FINGER FLEXION (DIP) 90 DEG		
		FIFTH FINGER EXTENSION (DIP) 0 DEG		
		HIP FLEXION 125 DEG		
		HIP EXTENSION 30 DEG		
		HIP ABDUCTION 45 DEG		
		HIP ADDUCTION 30 DEG		
		HIP INTERNAL ROTATION 45 DEG		
		HIP EXTERNAL ROTATION 45 DEG		
		KNEE FLEXION 135 DEG		
		KNEE EXTENSION 0 DEG		
		ANKLE PLANTARFLEXION 50 DEG		
		ANKLE DORSIFLEXION 20 DEG		
		ANKLE INVERSION 35 DEG		

(*continued*)

RANGE OF MOTION (*continued*)

RIGHT		NORMAL	LEFT	
PROM	AROM		PROM	AROM
		ANKLE EVERSION 20 DEG		
		GREAT TOE FLEXION (MTP) 45 DEG		
		GREAT TOE EXTENSION (MTP) 90 DEG		
		GREAT TOE FLEXION (IP) 90 DEG		
		GREAT TOE EXTENSION (IP) 0 DEG		
		SECOND TOE FLEXION (MTP) 40 DEG		
		SECOND TOE EXTENSION (MTP) 40 DEG		
		SECOND TOE FLEXION (PIP) 35 DEG		
		SECOND TOE EXTENSION (PIP) 0 DEG		
		SECOND TOE FLEXION (DIP) 30 DEG		
		SECOND TOE EXTENSION (DIP) 60 DEG		
		THIRD TOE FLEXION (MTP) 40 DEG		
		THIRD TOE EXTENSION (MTP) 40 DEG		
		THIRD TOE FLEXION (PIP) 35 DEG		
		THIRD TOE EXTENSION (PIP) 0 DEG		
		THIRD TOE FLEXION (DIP) 30 DEG		
		THIRD TOE EXTENSION (DIP) 60 DEG		
		FOURTH TOE FLEXION (MTP) 40 DEG		
		FOURTH TOE EXTENSION (MTP) 40 DEG		
		FOURTH TOE FLEXION (PIP) 35 DEG		
		FOURTH TOE EXTENSION (PIP) 0 DEG		
		FOURTH TOE FLEXION (DIP) 30 DEG		
		FOURTH TOE EXTENSION (DIP) 60 DEG		
		FIFTH TOE FLEXION (MTP) 40 DEG		
		FIFTH TOE EXTENSION (MTP) 40 DEG		
		FIFTH TOE FLEXION (PIP) 35 DEG		
		FIFTH TOE EXTENSION (PIP) 0 DEG		
		FIFTH TOE FLEXION (DIP) 30 DEG		
		FIFTH TOE EXTENSION (DIP) 60 DEG		
		TMJ PROTRACTION 1–3 CM		
		TMJ RETRACTION 0 CM		
		TMJ DEPRESSION 3–5 CM		
		TMJ ELEVATION 0 CM		
		TMJ LATERAL DEVIATION 1–3 CM		

Appendix C:

MUSCLE TESTING
SCALES[6,18,34,39,42,44,48,62,63,75,80,94106,115,149]

MANUAL MUSCLE TESTING

LOWMAN SCALELOVETT SCALE

5	NORMAL	Full range of motion against gravity. Muscle holds maximal resistance and has Good rebound.
4+	GOOD+	Full range of motion against gravity. Muscle holds maximal resistance, but slow Or no rebound is present.
4	GOOD	Full range of motion against gravity. Muscle gives eccentrically against maximal Resistance.
4−	GOOD−	Full range of motion against gravity. Muscle give with moderate resistance.
3+	FAIR+	Full range of motion against gravity. Muscle gives with minimal resistance.
3	FAIR	Full range of motion against gravity. Muscle cannot hold against any resistance.
3−	FAIR−	2/3 Range of motion against gravity only.
2+	POOR+	1/3 Range of motion against gravity only.
2	POOR	Positioned without gravity able to achieve full range of motion. No ROM against gravity.
2−	POOR−	Positioned without gravity able to achieve 2/3 full range of motion.
1+	TRACE+	Positioned without gravity able to achieve 1/3 full range of motion.
1	TRACE	Muscle tension palpated, but no range of motion is produced in a gravity free position.
0	NONE	No muscle tension is palpated.

351

DYSPNEA LEVELS

0 ABLE TO COUNT TO "15" EASILY IN 1 BREATH
1 ABLE TO COUNT TO "15" EASILY IN 2 BREATHS
2 ABLE TO COUNT TO "15" EASILY IN 3 BREATHS
3 ABLE TO COUNT TO "15" EASILY IN 4 BREATHS
4 UNABLE TO COUNT

PITTING EDEMA

1+ BARELY PERCEPTIBLE AFTER INDENTATION INTO TISSUE WITH INDEX FINGER
2+ <15 SECOND REBOUND AFTER INDENTATION INTO TISSUE WITH INDEX FINGER
3+ 15–30 SECOND REBOUND AFTER INDENTATION INTO TISSUE WITH INDEX FINGER
4+ >30 SECOND REBOUND AFTER INDENTATION INTO TISSUE WITH INDEX FINGER

REFLEXES

0 NO RESPONSE (A-REFLEXIA)
1 DECREASED RESPONSE (HYPO-REFLEXIA)
2 NORMAL RESPONSE
3 INCREASED RESPONSE (HYPER-REFLEXIA)
4 SPASTIC

BORG RATE PERCEIVED EXERTION SCALE

6
7 VERY, VERY LIGHT
8
9 VERY LIGHT
10
11 FAIRLY LIGHT
12
13 SOMEWHAT HARD

14
15 HARD
16
17 VERY HARD
18
19 VERY, VERY HARD
20

STATIC BALANCE

4 NORMAL   Can be challenged without the patient weight shifting.
3 GOOD   Can weight shift when challenged to maintain posture.
2 FAIR   Patient can assume and maintain posture, but not accept challenge.
1 POOR   Patient can assume but NOT maintain posture.
0 ABSENT   Cannot assume or maintain posture.

*note challenge is usually postural nudges

DYNAMIC BALANCE

4 NORMAL   No deficits, good balance responses bilaterally.
3 GOOD   Minimal risk for falls, patient self corrects instability.
2 FAIR   Moderate risk for falls, difficulty with self-correction.
1 POOR   High risk for falls, unable to self correct instability.
0 ABSENT   Needs full support for any movement.

Appendix D:

STANDARDIZED STRENGTH MEASUREMENTS [6,18,34,39,42,44,48,62,63,75,80,94106,115,149]

Grip Strength (Female, Units in Pounds of Force)

Age Group	Percentile 10th		Percentile 25th		Percentile 50th		Percentile 75th		Percentile 90th	
	R	L	R	L	R	L	R	L	R	L
20–24	48	41	55	49	62	57	70	64	77	71
25–29	46	39	53	47	61	55	68	62	75	70
30–34	45	38	51	46	60	54	67	61	74	68
35–39	43	36	50	44	58	52	65	60	72	67
40–44	41	35	48	43	56	50	64	58	71	65
45–49	40	33	47	41	55	49	62	57	69	64
50–54	38	32	45	40	53	48	60	55	67	62
55–59	37	30	44	38	51	46	59	54	66	61
60–64	35	29	42	37	50	45	57	52	64	59
65–69	33	27	40	35	48	43	55	51	63	58
70–74	32	26	39	34	46	41	54	50	61	56
75–79	30	24	37	32	45	40	52	48	60	55
80–84	29	23	36	31	43	39	50	46	58	54

Grip Strength (Male, Units in Pounds of Force)

Age Group	Percentile 10th		Percentile 25th		Percentile 50th		Percentile 75th		Percentile 90th	
	R	L	R	L	R	L	R	L	R	L
20–24	98	90	110	102	126	116	138	130	150	141
25–29	94	86	106	98	120	112	134	126	146	137
30–34	90	82	102	94	116	108	129	122	142	132
35–39	86	78	98	90	112	104	124	117	138	128
40–44	80	74	93	86	108	100	120	113	134	124
45–49	76	69	89	81	103	95	116	108	129	120
50–54	72	65	84	77	99	91	112	104	124	116
55–59	68	61	80	73	94	87	108	100	120	112
60–64	63	56	76	69	90	82	103	96	116	108

354

Age Group	Percentile 10th		Percentile 25th		Percentile 50th		Percentile 75th		Percentile 90th	
	R	L	R	L	R	L	R	L	R	L
65–69	59	52	71	65	86	78	98	92	111	104
70–74	54	48	66	60	81	74	94	88	106	100
75–79	50	44	62	56	76	70	90	84	102	96
80–84	46	40	58	52	72	66	85	80	98	91

PINCH STRENGTH

TIP PINCH–pinch ends of pinch meter between tips of thumb and index finger

MALE	AGE	AGE	AGE	AGE	AGE	AGE	AGE
	20 yrs	30 yrs	40 yrs	50 yrs	60 yrs	70 yrs	75+
Right	18#	18#	18#	18#	16#	14#	14#
Left	18#	18#	18#	18#	15#	13#	14#

FEMALE	AGE	AGE	AGE	AGE	AGE	AGE	AGE
	20 yrs	30 yrs	40 yrs	50 yrs	60 yrs	70 yrs	75+
Right	11#	13#	11#	12#	10#	10#	10#
Left	10#	12#	11#	11#	10#	10#	9#

LATERAL PINCH–pinch between pad of thumb and lateral surface of index finger

MALE	AGE	AGE	AGE	AGE	AGE	AGE	AGE
	20 yrs	30 yrs	40 yrs	50 yrs	60 yrs	70 yrs	75+
Right	26#	26#	26#	27#	23#	19#	20#
Left	25#	26#	25#	26#	22#	19#	19#

FEMALE	AGE	AGE	AGE	AGE	AGE	AGE	AGE
	20 yrs	30 yrs	40 yrs	50 yrs	60 yrs	70 yrs	75+
Right	18#	19#	17#	17#	15#	14#	13#
Left	16#	18#	16#	16#	14#	14#	11#

PALMER PINCH–pinch between pad of thumb and pad of index and middle finger

MALE	AGE	AGE	AGE	AGE	AGE	AGE	AGE
	20 yrs	30 yrs	40 yrs	50 yrs	60 yrs	70 yrs	75+
Right	27#	25#	24#	24#	22#	18#	19#
Left	26#	25#	25#	24#	21#	19#	18#

FEMALE	AGE	AGE	AGE	AGE	AGE	AGE	AGE
	20 yrs	30 yrs	40 yrs	50 yrs	60 yrs	70 yrs	75+
Right	17#	19#	17#	17#	15#	14#	12#
Left	16#	18#	17#	16#	14#	14#	12#

BIBLIOGRAPHY

1. Abraham, WM: Factors in delayed muscle soreness. Med Sci Sports 9:11, 1977.
2. Akeson, WH, et al: Effects of immobilization on joints. Clin Orthop Rel Res 219:28, 1987.
3. American College of Sports Medicine: Guidelines for Graded Exercise Testing and Exercise Prescription, ed 2. Lea and Febiger, Philadelphia, 1986.
4. American Physical Therapy Association: Standards of Practice for Physical Therapy, 2000.
5. Anderson B, Burke ER. Scientific, medical, & practical aspects of stretching. Clinics in Sports Medicine. 10(1):63–87, 1991.
6. Argur AM. Grant's Atlas of Anatomy. Baltimore, MD. Williams and Wilkins 1991.
7. Artal, R and Wiswell, R: Exercise in Pregnancy. Williams and Wilkins, Baltimore, 1986.
8. Barnes, W: Relationship between motor unit activation to muscular contraction at different contractile velocities. Phys Ther 60:1152, 1980.
9. Bennett, JG and Stauder, WT: Evaluation and treatment of anterior knee pain using eccentric exercise. Med Sci Sports 18:526, 1986.
10. Berkow R. The Merck Manual. Rathway, NJ: Merck & Co. Inc; 1992.
11. Blackburn, TA, McLeod, WD, White, B, and Wofford, L. EMG analysis of posterior rotator cuff exercises. Journal of Athletic Training. Vol. 25(1), 40–45, 1990.
12. Brar SP, Smith MB, Nelson LM, et al. Evaluation of treatment protocols on minimal to moderate spasticity in multiple sclerosis. Arch Phys Med Rehabil. 72(3):186–189, 1991.
13. Brotzman SB. Handbook of Orthopaedic Rehabilitation, St. Louis, MO: CV Mosby; 1996.
14. Byrnes WC, Clarkson PM. Delayed onset muscle soreness and training. Clinics in Sports Medicine. 5(3):605–612, 1986.
15. Campbell, D and Glenn, W: Rehabilitation of knee flexor and knee extensor muscle strength in patients with meniscectomies, ligamentous repairs and chondromalacia. Phys Ther 62:10, 1982.
16. Cerny K. Vastus medialis oblique/vastus lateralis muscle activity ratios for selected exercises in persons with and without patellar-femoral pain syndrome. Phys Ther. 75(8):672–684, 1995.
17. Chamberlain, G: Cyriax's friction massage: A review. JOSPT 4:16, 1982.
18. Chung KW. Gross Anatomy. Baltimore, MD. Williams and Wilkins 1991.
19. Cibulka MT, Martin DL. Evaluation and rehabilitation of injuries to the sacroiliac joint in the athlete. 1996 Sports Phys Ther Home Study Course.
20. Ciullo JV, Zarins B. Biomechanics of the musculotendinous unit: relation to athletic performance and injury. Clinics in Sports Medicine. 2(1):71–85, 1983.

21. Davies, GJ: A Compendium of Isokinetics in Clinical Usage and Rehabilitation Techniques, ed 4. S & S Publishing, LaCrosse, WI 1985.
22. Davies, GJ, Dickoff-Hoffman, S. Neuromuscular testing and rehabilitation of the shoulder complex. Journal of Orthopaedic and Sports Physical Therapy. Vol. 18(2) 449–458, August, 1993.
23. Delacerda FG. A comparative study of three methods of treatment for shoulder girdle myofascial syndrome. J Orthop Sports Phys Ther. 4:51–54, 1982.
24. DeLorme, TL and Watkins, A: Technics of progressive resistance exercise. Arch Phys Med Rehabil. 29:263, 1948.
25. DePalma, BF and Zelko, RR: Rehabilitation following anterior cruciate ligament surgery. Athl Train 21:200, 1986.
26. Fardy, P: Isometric exercise and the cardiovascular system. Phys Sports Med 9:43, 1981.
27. Fernhall B, Congdon K, Manfredi T. ECG response to water and land based exercise in patients with cardiovascular disease. J Cardiopulm Rehabil. 10:5–11, 1990.
28. Flynn TW, Soutas RW. Patellofemoral joint compressive forces in forward and backward running. J Orthop Sports Phys Ther. 21(5):277–282, 1995.
29. Fox, EL, Robinson, S, and Wiegman, D: Metabolic energy sources during continuous and interval running. J Appl Physiol 27:174, 1969.
30. Francabandera FL, Holland NJ, Wiesel-Levison P, et al. Multiple sclerosis rehabilitation: inpatient vs. outpatient. Rehabil Nurs. 13(5):251–253, 1988.
31. Francis, KT: Delayed muscle soreness: A review. JOSPT 5(1):10, 1983.
32. Garn, SN and Newton, RA: Kinesthetic awareness in subjects with multiple ankle sprains. Phys Ther 68:1669, 1988.
33. Garrett WE, Califf JC, Bassett FH. Histochemical correlates of hamstring injuries. J Sports Med. 12(2):98–102, 1984.
34. Gatorade Sports Science Institute. *www.gssiweb.com.* Chicago 1993–2003.
35. Gehlsen GM, Grigsby SA, Winant DM. Effects of aquatic fitness program on the muscular strength and endurance of patients with multiple sclerosis. Phys Ther. 64(5):653–657, 1984.
36. Gleim GW, Stachenfeld NS, Nicholas JA. The influence of flexibility on the economy of walking and jogging. J Orthop Res. 8(6):814–823, 1990.
37. Godges JJ, MacRae H, Engelke KA. Effects of exercise on hip range of motion, trunk muscle performance and gait economy. Phys Ther. 73(7):468–477, 1993.
38. Godges JJ, MacRae H, Longdon C, et al. The effects of two stretching procedures on hip range of motion and gait economy. J Orthop Sports Phys Ther. 10(9):350–357, 1989.
39. Gogia P. Clinical Orthopedic Tests, Tucson, AZ: Therapy Skill Builders, 1994.
40. Grana WA, Teague B, King M. An analysis of rotator cuff repair. Am J Sports Med. 22:585–588, 1994.
41. Guccione AA. Arthritis and the process of disablement. Phys Ther. 74(5):408–414, 1994.
42. Guyton AC. Textbook of Medical Physiology, Philadelphia, WB Saunders, 1991.
43. Hellebrandt, FA and Houtz, SJ: Mechanisms of muscle training in man: Experimental demonstration of the overload principle. Phys Ther Rev 36:371, 1956.

44. Hillegass EA, Sadosky HS. Essentials of Cardiopulmonary Physical Therapy. Philadelphia, PA: WB Saunders Co;1994.

45. Hislop, HJ and Perrine, J: The isokinetic concept of exercise. Phys Ther 47:114, 1967.

46. Hobbel SL, Rose DJ. The relative effectiveness of three forms of visual knowledge of results on peak torque output. J Orthop Sports Phys Ther. 18(5):601–605, 1993.

47. Hollis, M: Practical Exercise Therapy. Blackwell Scientific Publications, Oxford, 1976.

48. Hoppenfeld S. Physical Examination of the Spine and Extremities. New York, NY: Appleton & Lange;1976.

49. Hunter, JM (ed): Rehabilitation of the Hand. CV Mosby, St. Louis, 1980.

50. Hyde, SA: Physiotherapy in Rheumatology. Blackwell Scientific Publication, Oxford, 1980.

51. Iversen, LD and Clawson, DK: Manual of Acute Orthopedic Therapeutics, ed 2. Little, Brown and Company, Boston, 1982.

52. Jenkins, WL, Thackaberry, M, and Killian, C: Speed specific isokinetic training. JOSPT 6:181, 1984.

53. Jette AM, Smith K, Haley SM, Davis KD. Physical therapy episodes of care for patients with low back pain. Phys Ther. 74(2):101–109, 1994.

54. Johnson, BL, et al: A comparison of concentric and eccentric muscle training. Med Sci Sports 8(1):35, 1976.

55. Johnson CL. Physical therapists as scar modifiers. Phys Ther. 64(9):1381–1387, 1984.

56. Jones, H: The valsalva procedure: Its clinical importance to the physical therapist. J Am Phys Ther Assoc 45:570, 1965.

57. Judge JO, Underwood M, Gennosa T. Exercise to improve gait velocity in older persons. Arch Phys Med Rehabil. 74(4):400–406, 1993.

58. Kaplan, EG, et al: A triligamentous reconstruction for lateral ankle instability. J Foot Surg 23:24, 1984.

59. Kay, DB: The sprained ankle: Current therapy. Foot and Ankle 6:22, 1985.

60. Kealy GP, Jensen KT. Aggressive approach to physical therapy management of the burned hand. Phys Ther. 68(5):683–685, 1988.

61. Kellett KM, Kellett DA, Nordholm LA. Effects of an exercise program on sick leave due to back pain. Phys Ther. 71(4):283–291, 1991.

62. Kendall, FP, Muscles: Testing and Function. Williams & Wilkins, Baltimore, 1983.

63. Kessler, R and Hertling, D: Management of Common Musculoskeletal Disorders. Harper and Row, Philadelphia, 1983.

64. Kisner C, Colby LA. Therapeutic Exercise: Foundations and Techniques. Philadelphia, PA: FA Davis Co.;1990.

65. Knapik, JJ, Mawadsley, RH and Ramos, MU: Angular specificity and test mode specificity of isometric and isokinetic strength training. JOSPT 5:58, 1983.

66. Knight, KL: Knee rehabilitation by the daily adjustable progressive resistive exercise technique. Am J Sports Med 7:336, 1979.

67. Knight KL: Quadriceps strengthening with DAPRE technique: Case studies with neurological implications. Med Sci Sports Exerc 17:636, 1985.

68. Knuttgren, HG: Neuromuscular Mechanisms for Therapeutic and Conditioning Exercise. University Park Press, Baltimore, 1976.
69. Koch M, Gottschalk M, Baker DI, et al. An impairment and disability assessment and treatment protocol for community living elderly persons. Phys Ther. 74(4): 286–294, 1994.
70. Kottke FJ, Lehmann JF. Krusen's Handbook of Physical Medicine and Rehabilitation. Philadelphia, PA: WB Saunders Co.;1990.
71. Kopell, H and Thompson, W: Peripheral Entrapment Neuropathies, ed 2. Robert E Krieger, Huntington, NY 1976.
72. Koury MJ, Scarpelli E. A manual therapy approach to evaluation and treatment of a patient with a chronic lumbar nerve irritation. Phys Ther. 74(6):548–560, 1994.
73. Laird, CG and Rozier, CK: Toward understanding the terminology of exercise mechanics. Phys Ther 59:287, 1979.
74. Lattanza, L, Gray, GW, and Kantner, R: Closed vs open kinematic chain measurements of subtalar joint eversion: Implications for clinical practice. JOSPT 9:310, 1988.
75. Lehmkuhl LD, Smith LK. Brunnstrom's Clinical Kinesiology. 4th ed. Philadelphia, PA: F.A. Davis Co.;1983.
76. Lentell G, Hetherington T, Eagan J, Morgan M. The use of thermal agents to influence the effectiveness of a low-load prolonged stretch. J Orthop Sports Phys Ther. 16(5):200–207, 1992.
77. Lewis CB, Bottomley JM. Geriatric Physical Therapy. Norwalk, CT: Appleton and Lange;1994.
78. Lewis CL. Fitness for Kids with Down s Syndrome. Advance for PT. 2:53–55, 2000.
79. Lindh, M: Increase of muscle strength from isometric quadriceps exercise at different knee angles. Scand J Med 11:33, 1979.
80. Magee DJ. Orthopedic Physical Assessment. Philadelphia, PA: WB Saunders Co.;1992.
81. Maitland, GD: Peripheral Manipulation, ed 2. Butterworth, Boston, 1977.
82. Maitland, GD: Vertebral Manipulation, ed 4. Butterworth, Boston, 1977.
83. Malasanos L, Barkauskas V, Moss M, Stoltenberg-Allen K. Health Assessment. St. Louis, MO: CV Mosby Co.;1981.
84. Malone, T, Blackburn, T, and Wallace, L: Knee rehabilitation. Phys Ther 60: 1602, 1980.
85. Martin PE, Morgan DW. Biomechanical considerations for economical walking and running. Med Sci Sport Exerc. 24(4):467–474, 1991.
86. Mattsson E. Energy cost of level walking. Scand J Rehabil Med Suppl. 23:1–48, 1989.
87. Mattsson E, Brostrom LA, Borg J, Karlsson J. Walking efficiency before and after long-term muscle stretch in patients with spastic paresis. Scand J Rehabil Med. 22:55–59, 1990.
88. McConnell, JS. The management of chondromalacia patella: A long term solution. Australian Journal of Physiotherapy . 32(4):215–233.
89. McKenzie, R: The Lumbar Spine: Mechanical Diagnosis and Therapy. Spinal Publications, New Zealand, 1981.

90. McLaughlin HL: Rupture of the rotator cuff. J Bone Joint Surg 1962, 44A:979–983.
91. Muller, EA: Influence of training and inactivity on muscle strength. Arch Phys Med Rehabil 51:449, 1970.
92. Nerschel, R and Sobel, J: Conservative treatment of tennis elbow. Phys Sports Med 9(6):43, 1981.
93. Nichols DS, Glenn TM. Effects of aerobic exercise on pain perception affect, and level of disability in individuals with fibromyalgia. Phys Ther. 74(4):327–332, 1994.
94. Norkin, C, and Levangie, P: Joint Structure and Function: A Comprehensive Analysis. FA Davis, Philadelphia, 1983.
95. Noyes FR, Mangine RE, Barber SD. The early treatment of motion complications after reconstruction of the anterior cruciate ligament. Clin Ortho & Related Research. 277:217–228, 1992.
96. Oatis, CA: Biomechanics of the foot and ankle under static conditions. Phys Ther 68:1815, 1988.
97. O'Neil MB, Woodard M, Sosa V, et al. Physical therapy assessment and treatment protocol for nursing home residents. Phys Ther. 72(8):596–604, 1992.
98. Osternig LR, Robertson R, Troxel R, Hansen P. Muscle activation during proprioreceptive neuromuscular facilitation (PNF) stretching techniques. Am J Phys Med. 66(5):298–307, 1987.
99. Pace, JB, Nagle, D. Piriformis Syndrome. West J. Med. 124:435–439, June 1976.
100. Paris, SV: Mobilization of the spine. Phys Ther 59:988, 1979.
101. Penjabi, MM, Krag, MH, and Chung TQ: Effects of disc injury on mechanical behavior of the human spine. Spine 9:707, 1984.
102. Penny, JW and Welsh, MB: Shoulder impingement syndromes in athletes and their surgical management. Am J Sports Med 9:11, 1981.
103. Porterfield, JA: Dynamic stabilization of the trunk. JOSPT 6:271, 1985.
104. Richards CL, Malovin F, Dumas F. Effects of a single session of prolonged plantar flexion stretch on muscle activations during gait in spastic cerebral palsy. Scand J Rehabil Med. 23:103–111, 1991.
105. Richardson C, Hodges P. New Advances in Exercise to Rehabilitate Spinal Stabilisation. Spinal Pain Muscle Research Group, Queensland, Australia, 1996.
106. Richardson JK, Iglarsh ZA. Clinical Orthopaedic Physical Therapy. Philadelphia, PA: WB Saunders Co; 1994.
107. Rocobado, M: Temporomandibular Joint Dysfunctions. Workshop Miami, 1995.
108. Ruoti RG, Troup JT, Berger RA. The effects of nonswimming water exercises on older adults. J Orthop Sports Phys Ther. 19(3):140–145, 1994.
109. Sahrman, SA. Muscle Imbalances in the Orthopaedic and Neurologic Patient. World Confederation for Physical Therapy, Sydney Australia, 1987.
110. Sahrmann, SA: Diagnosis and treatment of muscle imbalances associated with musculoskeletal pain. APTA Conference, St. Louis, 1993.
111. Sapega, AA and Drillings, G: The definition and assessment of muscular power. JOSPT 5(1):7, 1983.
112. Saunders HD, Saunders R. Evaluation, Treatment and Prevention of Musculoskeletal Disorders. 3rd ed. Volume 1 Spine. Bloomington, MN: Educational Opportunities;1993.

113. Saunders HD, Saunders R. Evaluation, Treatment and Prevention of Musculoskeletal Disorders. 3rd ed. Volume 2 Extremities. Bloomington, MN: Educational Opportunities; 1993.

114. Sczepanski Tl, Gross MT, Duncan PW, Chandler JM. Effect of contraction type, angular velocity, and arc of motion on VMO:VL EMG ratio. J Orthop Sports Phys Ther. 14(6):256–265, 1991.

115. Scully RM, Barnes MR. Physical Therapy. Philadelphia, PA: JB Lippincott Co.; 1989.

116. Shelbourne KD, Nitz P. Accelerated rehabilitation after anterior cruciate ligament reconstruction. JOSPT 1992l15:256–264.

117. Simkin, PA: Tendinitis and bursitis of the shoulder, anatomy and therapy. Postgrad Med 73:177, 1983.

118. Smith CA. The warm–up procedure: to stretch or not to stretch. A brief review. J Orthop Sports Phys Ther. 19(1):12–17, 1994.

119. Smith, K: The thoracic outlet syndrome: A protocol of treatment. JOSPT 1:89, 1979.

120. Smith LL, Keating MN, Holbert D, et al: The effects of athletic massage on delayed onset muscle soreness, creatine kinase, and neutrophil count: a preliminary report. J Orthop Sports Phys Ther. 19:93–98, 1994.

121. Stenstrom CH. Radiologically observed progression of joint destruction and its relationship with demographic factors, disease severity, and exercise frequency in patients with rheumatoid arthritis. Phys Ther. 74(1):32–39, 1994.

122. Steward B, Woodman R, Hurlburt D. Fabricating a splint for deep friction massage. J Orthop Sports Phys Ther. 21(3):172–175, 1995.

123. Sullivan, P, Markos, P and Minor, M: An Integrated Approach to Therapeutic Exercise: Theory and Clinical Application. Reston Publishing Co., Reston, VA, 1982.

124. Svendsen, B, Moe, K, and Merritt, R: Joint Mobilization Laboratory Manual: Extremity Joint Testing and Selected Treatment Techniques. Bryn Mawr, CA, 1981.

125. Swaim K. An alternative therapy: Pilates method. PT Magazine. 10:55–58, 1993.

126. Taylor BF, Waring CA, Brashear TA: The effects of therapeutic application of heat or cold followed by static stretch on hamstring muscle length. J Orthop Sports Phys Ther. 21:283–286, 1995.

127. Tchow, D, et al: Pelvic-floor musculature exercises in treatment of anatomical urinary stress incontinence. Phys Ther 68:652, 1988.

128. Tesh, KM, Dunn JS, and Evans, JH: The abdominal muscles and vertebral stability. Spine 12:501, 1987.

129. Thomee, R, et al: Slow or fast isokinetic training after knee ligament surgery. JOSPT 8:475, 1988.

130. Thompson LV. Effects of age and training on skeletal muscle physiology and performance. Phys Ther. 74(1):71–80, 1994.

131. Threlkeld, JA and Currier, DP: Osteoarthritis: Effects on synovial joint tissues. Phys Ther 68:346, 1988.

132. Timm, KE: Investigation of the physiological overflow effect from speed specific isokinetic activity. JOSPT 9:106, 1987.

133. Timm KE. Evaluation procedures for spinal injuries specific to the athlete. 1996 Sports Phys Ther Home Study Course.

134. Timm, KE and Patch, DG: Case study: Use of Cybex II velocity spectrum in the rehabilitation of post surgical knees. JOSPT 6:347, 1985.

135. Tippett, SR: Closed chain exercises. Orthop Physical Therapy Clin. North America 1(2):253–286, 1992.

136. Touchet RH. Floating through pregnancy. Biomechanics. 9:87–90, 1995.

137. Umphred DA. Neurological Rehabilitation. 2nd ed. St. Louis, MO: CV Mosby Co.;1990.

138. Voss, DE, Ionta, MK and Myers BJ: Proprioceptive Neuromuscular Facilitation, ed 3. Harper and Row, New York, 1985.

139. Waddell, G: A new clinical model for the treatment of low back pain. Spine 12:632, 1987.

140. Wadsworth, CT: Frozen shoulder. Phys Ther 66:1878, 1986.

141. Wadsworth, CT: Manual Examination of the Spine and Extremities. Williams and Wilkins, Baltimore, 1988.

142. Wang RY. Effect of proprioceptive neuromuscular facilitation on the gait of patients with hemiplegia of long and short duration. Phys Ther. 74(12):1108–1115, 1994.

143. Watson CJ, Schenkman M. Physical therapy management of isolated serratus anterior muscle paralysis. Phys Ther. 75(3):194–201, 1995.

144. Wessling KC, DeVane DA, Hylton CR. Effects of static stretch verses static stretch and ultrasound combined on triceps surae muscle extensibility in healthy women. Phys Ther. 67(5):674–679, 1987.

145. Wilk KE, Andrews JR, Clancy WG. Quadriceps muscular strength after removal of the central third patellar tendon for contralateral anterior cruciate ligament reconstruction surgery: a case study. J Orthop Sports Phys Ther. 1993: 18(6): 692–697.

146. Wilk, KE, Voight, ML, Keims, MA, Gambetta, V, Andrews, AR, and Dillman, CJ. Stretch-shortening drills for the upper extremities: Theory and clinical application. Journal of Orthopaedic and Sports Physical Therapy. Vol 17(5) 225–239, May, 1993.

147. Wilk KE, Romaniello WT, Soscia SM, et al. The relationship between subjective knee scores, isokinetic testing, and functional testing in the ACL reconstructed knee. J Orthop Sports Phys Ther. 1994;20(2):60–74.

148. Wilkinson A. Stretching the truth. A review of the literature on muscle stretching. Australian Physiotherapy. 38(4):282–286, 1992.

149. Woodburne RT, et al. Essentials of Human Anatomy. New York, Oxford university Press. 1988.

150. Wright PC. Fundamentals of acute burn care and physical therapy management. Phys Ther. 64(8):1217–1231, 1984.

151. Zinowieff, AN: Heavy resistance exercise: The Oxford technique. Br J Phys Med 14:129, 1951.

INDEX

Commonly Overlooked Thoracic Spine
  Conditions, 204
Concept of Muscle Balance
  Strength Ratios, 20
Contraindications (Exercise)
  General, 23
  General Lower Extremity, 105
  General Spinal, 173
  General Upper Extremity, 35
  Joint Mobilizations, 297
  Massage, 323

D

Daily Adjustable Progressive Resistance
  Exercise (DAPRE), 15
Delayed Onset Muscle Soreness (DOMS), 17
DeLorme Technique, 15
Diagnoses, (*See* Common Diagnoses)
Documentation, 9

E

Effleurage Massage, 325
Elbow and Forearm
  Hypermobility Diagnoses and Proven
    Therapeutic Exercises, 72
  Hypomobility Diagnoses and Proven
    Therapeutic Exercises, 70
  Imbalances, 68
  Mobilizations, 303
  Neurovascular Diagnoses and Proven
    Therapeutic Exercises, 76
  Post Fracture/Surgical Diagnoses and
    Proven Therapeutic Exercises, 77
Exercise Argot, 21

F

Fatigue, 18
Friction Massage, 328
Fryette's Laws of Spinal Motion, 311
Fulling Massage, 326
Functional Position of the Hand, 82

G

General Research TEX Pearls, 25
General Treatment
  Considerations:
  Ankle/Foot, 153
  Diagnosis, 7

Elbow/Forearm, 67
Evaluation, 5
General Spinal, 175
Hip, 109
Joint Mobilization, 301
Knee, 131
Massage, 325
Patient, 8
Shoulder, 39
Spine
  Cervical, 186
  Lumbar, 225
  Thoracic, 204
  Sacral-Iliac, 225
Treatment, 8
Wrist/Hand, 81
Goals/Benefits (Exercise)
  General, 24
  General Lower Extremity, 107
  General Spinal, 175
  General Upper Extremity, 36
  Joint Mobilizations, 298
  Massage, 324

H

Hip
  General Considerations, 109
  Hypermobility Diagnoses and Proven
    Therapeutic Exercises, 115
  Hypomobility Diagnoses and Proven
    Therapeutic Exercises, 111
  Imbalances, 110
  Mobilizations, 307
  Neurovascular Diagnoses and Proven
    Therapeutic Exercises, 119
  Post Fracture/Surgical Diagnoses and
    Proven Therapeutic Exercises, 121

I

Indications (Exercise)
  General, 24
  General Lower Extremity, 106
  General Spinal, 174
  General Upper Extremity, 36
  Joint Mobilizations, 297
  Massage, 324
Isokinetic Exercise, 10
Isokinetic Endurance Protocol, 16
Isokinetic Strength Protocol, 16
Isometric Exercise, 9

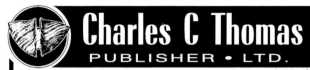
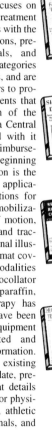
  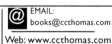 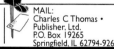